A MAN AG

MW00990372

Readers are encouraged to go to www.MissionPointPress.com to contact the author or to find information on how to buy this book in bulk at a discounted rate.

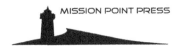

Published by Mission Point Press
2554 Chandler Rd.
Traverse City, MI 49696
(231) 421-9513
www.MissionPointPress.com

ISBN: 978-1-943995-55-4
Library of Congress Control Number: 2018932692

Printed in the United States of America.

A MAN AGAINST INSANITY

THE BIRTH OF DRUG THERAPY IN A RURAL MICHIGAN ASYLUM

PAUL DE KRUIF

MISSION POINT PRESS

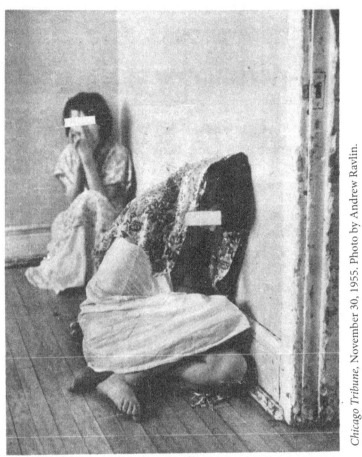

Chicago Tribune, November 30, 1955. Photo by Andrew Ravlin.

The disturbed ward is a frightening place. But now these lost souls have hope.

FOREWORD

A MAN AGAINST INSANITY describes the remarkable life
and career of Dr. John (Jack) Ferguson, a man who began his
medical career late in life with the simple goal of becoming a
simple country doctor.

But Dr. Ferguson was anything but a simple man, and this
book provides an insightful description of a tumultuous early
life that led to a relentless pursuit of goals motivated by an
insatiable need for approval. Despite repeated financial set-
backs, a divorce, a heart attack, a barbiturate addiction and
several psychiatric hospitalizations, Ferguson persevered
and eventually graduated medical school 20 years after he
first enrolled. He then realized his dream when he was hired
as the town doctor in a small, rural community. The dream
didn't last: after only one year, he abruptly abandoned his
position and collapsed into a fog of psychosis with grandiose
delusions, delusions that led to an attempt to poison his wife
and kill himself. Over the next 13 months, Ferguson would
be hospitalized three times as a barbiturate psychotic, finally
emerging as a "new man." Humbled and compassionate, Ferguson credited supportive psychotherapy and the warmth of
the hospital attendants with helping him find a new direction
for life—to serve psychiatric patients.

FOLLOWING THE CUSTOMS OF THE DAY, Ferguson
began training in psychosurgery. He mastered the transorbital lobotomy and developed an innovative technique that
drastically reduced surgical time and essentially eliminated

mortality. His success brought him to the Traverse City State Hospital, where 500 surgical lobotomies were planned. He never performed a single one. Instead, he embarked on a completely new therapeutic direction—chemistry and love.

Aware of the advances in the chemical treatment of schizophrenia, Ferguson began his "lone wolf" research on the 1000 female State Hospital patients assigned to him. Initially, he employed the tranquillizers Serpasil and Thorazine, then added an analeptic, Ritalin, to moderate the side effects. Ferguson's staff of 107 nurses was responsible for painstakingly cataloging behavioral changes and adjusting medication accordingly—observation being the only mechanism available at that time to evaluate change—while also providing comfort and encouragement. Ferguson would say, "We don't treat the disease, we treat the sick people." This balancing technique and the trial and error research method eventually liberated hundreds of women from decades of psychotic isolation in the locked hospital seclusion wards.

AUTHOR DE KRUIF'S STYLE provides an intriguing snapshot into the cultural mindset of the 1950s. The fact that Ferguson's initial research involved only female patients will not be lost to contemporary readers. Nonetheless, the improvement in functioning that Ferguson's chemical cocktails brought to people diagnosed with schizophrenia gained him national recognition and his results were widely replicated. As one colleague was quoted, "We can now talk directly to the person behind the schizophrenia."

Over time, Ferguson's dream that medication would allow the family physician to manage symptoms of schizophrenia became a reality. Thirty-two years after the publication of

A Man Against Insanity, Traverse City State Hospital closed its doors for the last time.

A MAN AGAINST INSANITY is a must-read for all students in the helping professions. Author DeKruif provides a fascinating overview of the scientific method and the state of psychiatric care from the early to mid-20th century, beginning with William Lorenz's 1916 proclamation that "insanity is chemical." Throughout the book, DeKruif charts the slow but steady course of scientific discovery, from the brief glimmers of normality triggered by sodium cyanide to the profoundly calming effects of the powdered root from India, *Rauwolfia serpentina,* the forerunner of the tranquillizer, Chlorpromazine.

A Man Against Insanity is an intriguing story about scientific discovery and the Northern Michigan physician who prevailed over personal adversity to lead in the development of modern psychopharmacology.

—*Michael J. Sullivan LMSW*
Family Psychotherapist

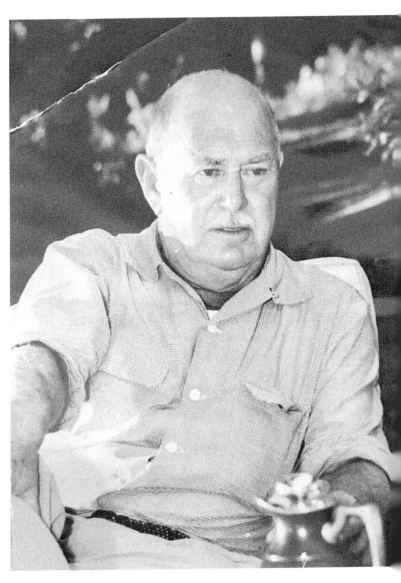

Paul De Kruif. (Photo courtesy of Susan Joyce)

PREFACE

IN 1957, DWIGHT EISENHOWER WAS PRESIDENT. *The Bridge on the River Kwai* and *12 Angry Men* were the movies people were talking about. Gas was around 24 cents per gallon, the Soviet Union launched Sputnik, and Michigan's Mackinac Bridge opened to traffic for the first time.

In other Michigan news, a book published by noted microbiologist turned author, Paul de Kruif, brought international fame to a small-town "country doctor" who worked at the Traverse City State Hospital. *A Man Against Insanity* focused on Dr. Jack Ferguson and his miracle therapy—using modern drugs and what he called "tender loving care"—for treating the mentally ill.

In 1957, any form of psychological abnormality, from schizophrenia and chronic depression to intellectual disability and age-induced dementia, could land a person in a state-sponsored psychiatric hospital where straightjackets, lobotomies and electroshock therapy were the go-to treatments of the day. Movies like *The Snake Pit* —a 1948 drama based on the real-life story of a woman who finds herself in an insane asylum—exposed some of these horrors. Americans began talking more about mental health reform, especially in the early 1950s, when chemists began to experiment with so-called "chemical restraints"—tranquilizers and drugs that could calm imbalances in the brain and soothe people with bipolar and psychotic disorders.

Drugs such as lithium, chlorpromazine (discovered in 1950 and eventually sold in America under the trade name, Thorazine) and the psycho-stimulant Ritalin (approved by the FDA in 1955) offered promise in treating the mentally ill, but they were hardly a one-size-fits-all cure that doctors had long sought.

Dr. Jack Ferguson, a lobotomy expert who had figured out a way to complete the operation in roughly three minutes, came to northern Michigan in 1954 to perform 500 lobotomies on so-called incurably insane patients at the Traverse City State Hospital.

"He never did get around to even the first one," reported Norma Lee Browning in the February 24, 1957, edition of the *Chicago Tribune*. "Instead, with an unscientific combination of chemicals plus love, he pierced the veil of insanity in one of the boldest, most bizarre and awesome experiments ever tried in a mental institution." Today, doctors routinely combine various drugs to achieve a desired effect. But in the mid-1950s, the idea was radical stuff.

Ferguson was also a complicated and controversial character. A considerable portion of de Kruif's *A Man Against Insanity* examines Ferguson's long and unconventional path to becoming a doctor, his personal battle with drug addiction and the health and emotional problems that led to repeated psychotic breakdowns. Over a 22-year span, Ferguson was taken into custody and hospitalized five times for drug addiction and concern for his mental health. In *A Man Against Insanity*, de Kruif captures the natural impact that the experience on the other side of the psychiatric fence—as a patient in a locked ward for the suicidal and paranoid disturbed—had on Ferguson's outlook and life's work.

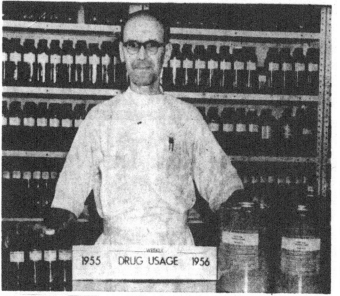

Chillicothe Gazette, February 27, 1957.

Barney B. Palkovacs, chief pharmacist at the Chillicothe VA Hospital, gives a graphical illustration of the use being made there of tranquilizing agents. In the four bottles are a total of 2000 Thorazine tablets which represents the average amount used per week in 1955. In the two cans are 10,000 Thorazine tablets, the average weekly consumption in 1956.

By 1954, Ferguson had fully recovered. But his checkered past and lack of psychiatric credentials—Ferguson was a general practitioner, not a licensed psychiatrist—had colleagues constantly questioning whether "Ferguson therapy" was pure genius or a hoax.

Ferguson found an ally in Zeeland, Michigan, native Paul de Kruif, who had spent his entire career explaining advances in science that could help common men. De Kruif began his vocation at the University of Michigan, obtaining a PhD. in microbiology. After graduation, he joined the military service, first as a private on the Pancho Villa Expedition in Mexico, and then as an officer in the Sanitary Corps during World War I, where he had occasion to meet many leading French scientists of the day.

In 1925, de Kruif assisted Sinclair Lewis in the research for his Pulitzer Prize-winning novel about the state of medicine in the U.S. during the 1920s, *Arrowsmith*, for which he received 25 percent of royalties. The very next year de Kruif published his own book, *Microbe Hunters*, which became a bestseller and still remains on recommended reading lists for phycians and scientists.

De Kruif supported the belief that healthcare should be made available to everyone, regardless of their ability to pay for treatments and services —something *Detroit Free Press* science writer Boyce Rensberger pointed out was "tantamount to treason among members of the medical community" in the 1950s, particularly the American Medical Association, which considered de Kruif a communist. In the words of Rensberger, de Kruif "fought an economic system that at the time withheld modern medicine's benefit for all but the wealthy."

Ferguson, on the other hand, was a quirky and unconventional visionary who perfected the lobotomy, then disavowed it. Equally, he saw solitary confinement and straightjackets as things of the past. His beliefs resonated with Americans, and his track record of saving so-called incurables—the long-term catatonic and violent maniacs in the locked, forgotten halls of the Traverse City State Hospital—further inspired a movement that wanted to see more oversight of mental hospitals and, ultimately, a better system of care and treatment aimed at returning loved ones to normal life. Ferguson believed his work could one day lead to the closing of state mental institutions, and that family doctors—once supplied with modern drugs and the knowledge of how to use them—could be the new frontline of mental health care.

For better or worse, Ferguson would never live to see his dreams come to fruition. On March 1, 1968, Ferguson—then age 59 and serving as the geriatric program director—died of a heart attack while trying to direct traffic after a minor fire broke out at the Traverse City State Hospital. Paul de Kruif died in 1971 at his beachfront home near Holland, Michigan. At 80 years old, he authored fourteen books over his five-decade writing career.

A MAN AGAINST INSANITY was first published in 1957 and rediscovered nearly 60 years later by pure serendipity. Marlas Hanson at the Traverse City Area District Library mentioned it to Anne Stanton of Mission Point Press, publisher of *How Thin the Veil*, a 1952 book that also took place at the Traverse City State Hospital. Hanson said De Kruif's book was even more deserving of a second life, as it told the story of a family doctor determined to help the comatose, violent and mostly forgotten patients though experimental drug therapy.

Luckily, the story could still be told; Mission Point Press worked with the De Kruif family to help it secure the rights from the original publisher, which had let the book go out of print. After an edit—for length and readability—and a redesign, the book is reborn here, in this new edition.

—Bob Butz, editor

A MAN AGAINST INSANITY

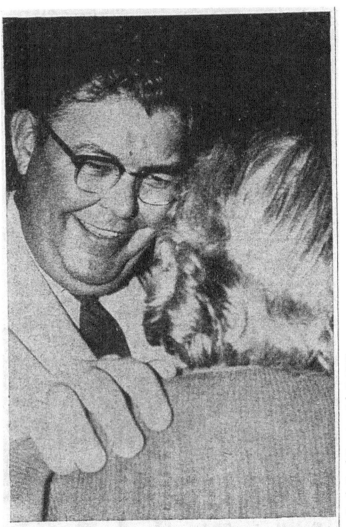

—Grand Rapids Press Photo.

Dr. John Ferguson mixes wonder drugs with "tender loving care" in revolutionizing the recovery of mental patients at the Traverse City state hospital. Here he talks with one of his patients who, like himself, knows first hand what it means to lose one's mind.

A NEW TYPE OF DOCTOR

B Y PROFESSION, JACK FERGUSON is a medical doctor, and his specialty is trying to help crazy people. But he thinks of himself simply as a general practitioner, a family physician, which indeed he was only six years ago until, in 1950, Ferguson was locked up in a mental hospital.

But eventually (and the precise medical explanation of how this transpired is not clear), he recovered. He came back to a steady, cool-headed sanity he had never experienced before. With the knowledge of what it truly means to be psychotic, he set off on an adventure against the insanity of others. Using new neuro-chemical medicines, he began treating many patients who were thought to be hopelessly crazy, and his results are remarkable.

Some regard Jack Ferguson as that new type of doctor, the chemical clinician, a futuristic character who believes that disease is chemical and more or less chemically reversible, correctable, and—maybe—curable. But the chemical clinician is only one part of this man. He combines his keen clinical intuition with another characteristic that is totally unscientific—love. Ferguson is a minister of tender loving care, which he lavishes impartially upon those who cannot live with themselves or others, upon those who are sinful or criminal, and those in trouble or sorrow. For him, there are no bad people; there are only sick people.

So Jack Ferguson is a new type of doctor. Call him "a chemical family doctor." He's no psychiatrist of the eminence of the Menninger brothers, who today are to psychiatry as the Mayo brothers were to surgery. Like the humble worker in the vineyard, Ferguson is a simple, medical bench worker, a natural caregiver with Dostoevskian insight into the human heart. In other words, he's a natural—a simple doctor with a serene disregard for scientific authority and a left-handed originality rare in the medical field nowadays.

THE TIME IS THE LATE 1950s, when it is evident that Ferguson's radical vision—blending the scientific AND spiritual to help crazy people—is as bold and beautiful as any I've known. And then there is the dark and bizarre life history of the man himself.

My interest in Ferguson, and what makes him tick, is linked to my homesickness for my own lost times. The old microbe hunters were my first heroes—rough-hewn, isolated geniuses like dry-goods merchant Antony van Leeuwenhoek, and Robert Koch, the dauntless little country doctor. They both had the integrity to report only what they saw in nature with their own eyes.

Jack Ferguson is a little like them, which is rare. As lab buildings get bigger and bigger, as the richer and richer money grants pay scientists to try to discover what they are told to find, searchers like Ferguson are harder and harder to find.

This is not meant in criticism; it's the way it is today in science. But this way is certainly not Jack Ferguson's. He does not try to bore deep into the scientific unknown, but stays shallow, on the surface, just watching with sharp eyes and reporting how new chemicals may change human vagaries.

Ferguson has another quirk: he genuinely believes his efforts are helping to make a different world, a new world, a wonderful world for us to live in. In that way he is like Pasteur, who said, "It is in the power of man to make parasitic maladies disappear from the face of the globe." That wasn't science. It was pure Beethoven, a trumpet blast of hope.

Since Ferguson is old-fashioned, his experimental setup in this era of super-gadgets is hardly inspiring. His laboratory is only the sadly sinister mental wards, the locked wards of the 3,000-bed Traverse City State Hospital. His apparatus? Only his own eyes and hands, plus the hands and eyes of more than 100 nurse attendants, who are a wonderful help to him because, so he says proudly, "They all have a high-school education or its equivalent."

His modest experiments amount only to Ferguson and his nurse attendants following the negligible, or eerie, often amazing neuropharmacology medicines now being cooked up by hundreds of organic chemists in dozens of laboratories on both sides of the Atlantic.

Ferguson and the sharp eyes of his nurses record whether or not these new medicines work a stimulating or calming chemistry on hundreds of confused, addled, suspicious, withdrawn, babbling, wildly screaming, sometimes violent beings—all of them thought to be demented past the point of no return.

And the result?

"With our present knowledge of these new drugs," says Ferguson, "there is no abnormal behavior that we cannot control or change for the better."

"Only by your knowledge of the new drugs?" I asked him.

Jack Ferguson's round face glowed red.

"Of course not," he admitted. "These chemicals only *start* them back to reality. It's the tender loving care of our nurse attendants, reassuring them they can again be human, that brings them back—many of them all the way."

Through the strange story that follows, remember the secret of Ferguson's work is only partly scientific. In other words, it is chemical—plus Ferguson.

SOME SCIENTIFIC CRITICS may smile at Ferguson's apparent shallowness, his belief that insanity, delinquency, un-respectability and evil conduct are best understood as "abnormal behavior." For this belief he has precedents.

Medicine men since the beginning of human record have tried to incant abnormal behavior out of mankind. Jailers have tried to drive it out by torture and death. Holy men, religious preachers and prophets had some success in admonishing abnormal behavior away by their example and teachings. Psychiatrists try to persuade abnormal behavior out of sufferers bereft of reason. Physicians chemically or electrically shock normal behavior into people by sending them into shattering convulsions. Neurosurgeons calm many insane people by slashing nerves in their brains after boring through their skulls or gouging through their eye sockets with a tool similar to an ice pick. And, when they're successful, what is the one proof for the effectiveness of all the above?

Only "better behavior," the very outcome Ferguson is after.

But Ferguson is perhaps different from his predecessors in his deep-down dissatisfaction. The family doctor in him revolts at the terror of shock treatment and the mutilating barbarity of ice picks rammed above the eyes to stir round in a patient's brain. He knows it's necessary. He knows this savage science testifies to the despair of men who fight severe mental illness. But Jack Ferguson knows, too, that these ferocious therapies can't be the sole answer to the fight against insanity in which all doctors, not just psychiatrists and surgeons, must have their part.

By the way these treatments helped some seemingly incurable psychotics, Ferguson learned even the worst behavior may be reversible. He was inspired by individual cases like this one: a woman, stark-staring mad, dying in the dementia of pellagra[1], was given a few massive shots of the B vitamin niacin, and with a clear head went home a week later. Her insanity had been due to the lack, the deficiency, of just one organic compound.

Unfortunately, not all mental sickness can be that simple. Unlike the fading menace of disease caused by microbes, insanity is on the upswing. Yet Ferguson always found optimism—something not shared by everyone in the medical community.

"If chemists could give Ferguson a medicine that would empty our hospital in a week," acting superintendent Dr. M. M. Nickels once said, "we'd be full up again in a couple of months."

Nickels was trying to point out the unfortunate backlog of the insane who were not yet institutionalized. To this, Ferguson only chuckled at his chief's pessimism. He repeated his confident claim.

---

1 A disease caused by low levels of niacin and marked by dementia, diarrhea and dermatitis—"the three Ds". Left untreated, pellagra can be fatal.

"There's no abnormal behavior that we cannot now control or change for the better," he said.

Despite his pessimism, "Dr. Nick" was immensely proud of Ferguson. He knew that hundreds of formerly hopeless patients were presently leaving for home, and that over half of the 1,000 patients under Ferguson's service could go home—if they were wanted or had homes to go to.

"Sure, there are more crazy people outside than inside mental hospitals," Ferguson once said to me. "But pretty soon our general practitioners will know how to keep them from coming here at all."

Like Pasteur, here was a new man of medicine with an illusion, an impossible dream. I felt sorry for him. How could a family doctor ever hope to stop insanity in its tracks, a task of which professional psychiatrists had failed? Ferguson didn't even have his diploma as a neuropsychiatric specialist.

Ferguson, the man, seemed as if he was fresh off a Hoosier farm. He didn't spell too well. His grammar left much to be desired. Culturally uncouth and—for a man already 47 years old—his academic position (a lowly resident at the Traverse City State Hospital in Michigan) was not impressive. He was just an obscure general practitioner who believed that family doctors like himself might one day be able to help solve medicine's most illusive problem.

UP UNTIL RECENTLY, Ferguson had been a rolling stone. Before getting into medicine, he had been a steel-mill cinder-snapper, a locomotive fireman on the Monon Railroad, a bartender, an insurance salesman and a whiskey peddler who had himself done several stretches in a mental institution. Along with 160,000 mainly anonymous Americans, he did have his medical degree, but it had taken him 18 years of his grown-up life to earn it.

The circumstances of Ferguson being institutionalized were intriguing. After obtaining his M.D. degree at age 40, he had a year of general internship followed by a year and a half of phenomenal success as a country doctor. Then, Ferguson had what he described as a "blow-up." The "blow-up" led to him being confined to a locked ward in a mental hospital.

But Jack Ferguson intrigued me, not only for his present work, but as a man unafraid of his troubled past. One conversation stands out when I initially expressed interest in writing a book about his work:

"If you're going to write about my work, you'd better know what's been bad about me," he said. "Among other things, I've been a barbiturate addict."

Ferguson spoke with a bemused, almost serene look of detachment on his face, as if he were speaking about another man.

"They carried me to the hospital, higher than a kite, and dangerous," Ferguson explained. "I was having hallucinations in Technicolor. I'd tried to kill myself, and my wife, Mary."

Because of his own experience, Ferguson knew what it meant to be insane—seemingly beyond the point of no return. Now he was taking advantage of a rare opportunity to investigate mental troubles at the obscure Traverse City State Hospital—a beautiful, sprawling complex in northern Michigan best known for its "work is therapy" philosophy. Because he was not focused on scientific research or sponsored by biased research underwriters who expected certain outcomes, he had as good a chance as any man to battle the world's aberrant behavior. Maybe better.

IN THE AUTUMN OF 1955, Ferguson began to show me how he was attacking the problem by boiling all mental illness down to one thing—abnormal behavior. Ferguson, of course, knows about schizophrenias and their sub-classified catatonias, hebephrenias, dissociations and paranoias; he can recite the difference between a reactive and endogenous depression and tell how these differ from a true involutional melancholia and the depressed phase of a genuine manic-depressive psychosis. In his work, however, he sees this jargon as something of a distraction. He would rather focus on the thing that results: the abnormal behavior that sends people to mental hospitals and drives family doctors to despair.

Jack Ferguson—for all his gentle manner of talking, his cherubic smile—became a medical desperado of sorts. To truly test if his theories worked, he knew he must work with the worst of the worst. For his experiments, he decided to delve deep into the forgotten locked wards of the state hospital where patients only "existed;" whom staff referred to as the "cats and dogs;"the seemingly incurable psychotics who proved resistant to all treatment and were far beyond hope.

Among the more than 1,000 patients under Ferguson's care were some early psychotics—the type that might well be helped by insulin or electro-shocks. But Ferguson took special interest in using his "chemicals AND love approach" on the abandoned wretches of the locked wards, and it's this fact that is, perhaps, the ultimate insight into the character and motive of Jack Ferguson.

Ferguson has many examples of his new chemicals plus tender loving care approach reversing the fate of patients deemed hopeless. And he believes his methods have a wider application—that perhaps someday his prescription for wellness might find itself in the hands of family doctors.

INSANITY IS CHEMICAL

BNORMAL BEHAVIOR.

Could the key to healing the minds of the so-called incurable really be so simple? Ferguson seemed to think so. On my very first visit to the Traverse City State Hospital, we spoke about the subject at length.

"Why are all these patients in this hospital?" he asked. "What do *you* think they're sent here for?"

"Why, because they're psychotic," I answered. "They're schizophrenics or paranoids or manic depressives or melancholics—"

"Take it easy with the big words," Ferguson broke in, smiling at my array of psychiatric terms. He pushed a pile of carbon copies of complaints that had led to commitment across the desk. "Take a look," he continued, "and see how wrong you are."

I thumbed through these terse records of family tragedy, a sad parade of people and problems:

"She keeps tearing her clothes off of her."
"We have to feed her every mouthful she eats."
"She doesn't know where the bathroom is."
"We try hard but we can't keep her clean."
"We're afraid she's going to set the house afire."
"She's always screaming and hollering."

"She's mean. She abuses us. She attacks us. We're afraid she'll kill us."

Ferguson watched me as I read and, when he decided I'd finally seen enough, he broke in,

"You see, it's simply their abnormal behavior that brings them here."

"But on their charts, it says they're schizophrenic, et cetera," I protested.

"That's for the records, the statistics," said Ferguson. "Pinning a big word on a patient as a diagnosis," he went on, "that doesn't help me one damn bit to get them better."

This was Ferguson's grammatically incorrect defiance of the first law of scientific medicine: that you must call a disease by its Greek or Latin name to treat it scientifically. It bothered me, this super-simplicity of Ferguson's, and it must have shown on my face.

"Maybe we're not scientific here," he said. "I know we're different than they are in the big medical schools. We don't treat *diseases*—we try to treat sick people."

DRIVING BACK HOME to Wake Robin after my meeting, I kept thinking about something else Ferguson said: "There's a lot more to mental illness than this abnormal behavior we're trying to treat here."

Yes, I wondered, but how much more? How much more that you can pin down as fact agreed to by honest and accurate men? How much more that you can get a-hold of like the way you can grip this big table on which I write?

Mulling this over took me back to almost forty years, to 1916 and the small but important discovery of a man—Dr. William F. Lorenz. A tough and wise physician, now living, actively, in retirement in the backwoods of north Wisconsin. Lorenz was then a professor of neuropsychiatry at the University of Wisconsin. I knew the man as a Brooklyn-born German with a faint New York accent. Lorenz had the square jaw, square head and the cold, farseeing eyes of a tank general. An "organicist," in the world of psychiatry, Lorenz was another doctor only interested in tangible facts, not in large words that may mean 50 different things to 50 people.

The ever-humble Lorenz always said that his important "observation"—he never called it a discovery—came very much as a surprise. Yet, what Lorenz saw that day 40 years ago not only justified but predicted today's astounding chemical fight against insanity.

ONE DAY EARLY IN HIS CAREER, Lorenz had been asked by his friend Dr. Arthur S. Loevenhart, the late great pharmacologist, to bring him a mental patient with a mind so far gone that he was no more than a vegetable. As part of his study on the action of sundry chemicals that might affect breathing when they were injected into the blood, Loevenhart was looking for a test subject so utterly mindless, so oblivious, that there'd be no so-called "psychological" effect, no deeper breathing at the moment the needle went into the patient's vein, before the chemical itself was injected.

Lorenz had just the patient—a man who for years was a victim of dementia praecox, the old-fashioned name for a bunch of assorted insanities that now go by the newfangled name of "schizophrenia." This man who Lorenz brought to Loevenhart was mute, rigid, with eyes either shut or staring blankly. He had no contact with reality. He was a full-blown example of mental deterioration, implying a degeneration that was advanced and irreparable. In short, this poor man had lost his mind for keeps.

So one day after bringing the patient to Loevenhart, Lorenz watched as a small, perfectly safe amount of sodium cyanide was injected into an arm vein of this mentally ill human being. It went exactly as the doctor expected: the patient didn't bat an eye or move a muscle until the cyanide took hold in the respiratory center of his brain. The patient began breathing deep, deeper and faster, and Dr. Loevenhart delighted as he monitored the breathing until suddenly the patient seemed to snap awake.

"Hello," the man said.

As this seemingly stupid, years-long mute patient breathed deeper, he also arose out of his supposed deterioration and looked at Bill Lorenz with a gleam of light in eyes that had been for so long blank and dead. Lorenz saw intelligence reborn in this man whose mind was assumed to be gone for good.

The man smiled at Lorenz, and, when asked, gave his own name clearly.

"Where are you?" asked Lorenz.

"At the Wisconsin Psychiatric Institute," said the man.

For three, four, five minutes, the dumb man talked with not a hint of ever having been off the beam. But just as suddenly, as the cyanide effect wore off, the patient's breathing quieted and his conversation slowly trailed off into a mumble. His eyes, once again, went blank.

On the surface, it was really nothing—a five-minute "cure" of incurable insanity. But to Lorenz it opened a new world. For a moment, he had seen a veil lifted, chemically, to reveal sanity—latent—but sanity existing in a brain that was supposed, by all clinical experience, to be dead and gone.

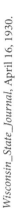

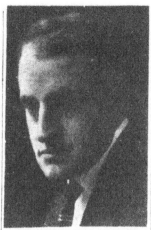

DR. WILLIAM F. LORENZ

WHAT LORENZ SAW 40 YEARS AGO was no happenstance, because again and again he repeated the experiment on this same patient and other hopeless schizophrenics: a shot of sodium cyanide; the bringing on of deeper breathing; and then a dawning and high noon of clear-headedness. After a few minutes, there was twilight and black night again as the deep breathing died down. For the world's millions of severely mentally sick, it meant nothing—after all, you couldn't keep people sane on shots of cyanide.

But for Lorenz, this forgotten experiment was tantalizing, suggesting that a slight shift in the oxidations in brain cells, a chemical shift brought on by this deeper breathing, could make temporary order in the most disordered chemical housekeeping of the sickest brain. Insanity? It's a chemical shift from the brain's normal sanity. In a most insane human being, this sanity is there, but masked.

Insanity is chemical.

This became Lorenz's lifelong hope. And it was what Jack Ferguson meant when he said there was more to mental illness than abnormal behavior.

VERY SOON AFTER his completely impractical discovery of five-minute lucidity in a man who had spent years in incurable insanity, Bill Lorenz got embroiled in the general

13

insanity of World War I and its aftermath. He had to put his hopeful theory on ice for years.

Meanwhile, the more and more prevailing doctrine in many medical schools was that insanity is not chemical. The cause, said the mental moguls, is *psychogenic*. This is a big-word way to say that the cause of a sick brain is only in your mind.

But what *is* the mind? It's in no sense tangible. The mind is nothing you can hear or touch or smell or feel or see. It isn't chemical; it isn't physical or in any sense material; it has no location in the body. Your mind is a vague, constantly shifting and fluctuating sum total of the brain's activities.

So if the cause of a sick brain is only in your mind, this was moonshine to such a matter-of-fact man as Bill Lorenz.

For some years, Lorenz brooded alone, haunted by the fact of the five-minute lucid interval in the doomed, incurably insane. Then Arthur Loevenhart, his old partner in that first sodium cyanide experiment, came to his rescue. "Maybe anything that'll stimulate breathing will do the same trick," Loevenhart wondered. "Maybe do it even better than our cyanide."

In 1928, Lorenz and Loevenhart went to work again and eventually proved that merely inhaling mixtures of carbon dioxide and oxygen through an anesthetic mask brought on spells of lucidity to certain muddled, deeply-depressed lunatics and catatonic schizophrenics. Even more exciting was that this lucidity lasted much longer than the one that followed sodium cyanide.

Among certain—but by no means all—catatonics, this carbon dioxide-oxygen inhalation worked weird wonders. For as long as 30 minutes, the supposedly incurable patient unwound and let go. Their pale, muddy faces turned a healthy pink. Their eyes that had been clamped shut opened with a spark as they saw their darkness change to a world that was bright and sane. They became vivacious. They winked at Bill Lorenz as if to say, "And *you* thought I was crazy."

"Their psychotic reactions seem to be entirely absent," wrote Lorenz. "The patients' thoughts and interests are amazingly normal."

NOW THAT LORENZ had shown that he could get some crazy people back on the beam for as long as 30 minutes by these inhalations, he set up what seemed to be a more hopeful, as well as reasonable, experiment. If the inhalations made people sane and rational, might they be accessible in this brief period to lecturing and questioning about what, in the beginning, had driven them crazy?

"These patients revealed past experiences that could well account for their deep depressions," said Lorenz, who began experiments in psychotherapy aimed at persuading his momentarily sane patients to stay that way, permanently.

It shouldn't fail, Lorenz reasoned, because the idea was so reasonable. The carbon dioxide-oxygen inhalations gave him time for a 30-minute sermon on how wrong his patients' minds had been to drive their brains insane. And the patients, breathing deeply, agreed absolutely, admitting they had been really foolish to have gone crazy. But always and eventually, the patients would quiet. They would again begin to mumble, look pale and gloomy, their faces went blank. It was as if their brief spate of mental clarity had only been something in Lorenz's own crazy dream.

"Psychotherapy?" wrote Lorenz. "We found its therapeutic results to be negligible. No lasting benefits were observed."

So again, for the world's millions of mentally sick, this lucid interval, though longer, meant nothing. You couldn't keep them sane by organizing them into brigades to inhale carbon dioxide-oxygen every other half-hour, 24 hours daily, 365 days a year.

Still, I understand how Bill Lorenz's pathetic little discovery gave me confidence and hope. As Jack Ferguson says: "Today, it opened a door to reality."

Lorenz was tough and skeptical. Ferguson is enthusiastic. But the two of them as experimenters are like two peas in a pod. Ferguson believes that there's more to mental illness than the abnormal behavior he is treating, but Lorenz had begun to find what this "more" actually is—namely, the secret chemistry of a sick brain. He had begun to uncover this secret by following the simple surface facts of the abnormal behavior of the insane.

IN 1929, A YEAR AFTER his initial inhalation experiments, one of Lorenz's associates revealed another secret of mental illness, deep below the surface of abnormal behavior.

It started with a patient, a woman laying mute and rigid at the Wisconsin Psychiatric Institute. Nurses couldn't get through her fog when they tried to make her eat; she had to be tube-fed to be kept alive. She couldn't take care of her natural needs. She lay rigid in a curled-up position. Lorenz's assistant, Dr. William Bleckwenn, was trying this and that to relieve the terrible tenseness of the woman.

Dr. Bleckwenn was only trying to make her a bit more comfortable—he hoped for nothing more. Snowing her under with a big injection of sodium amytal, he watched as she went limp. She relaxed into something far deeper than mere sleep, so deep that her reflexes were gone. The only signs of life were an almost imperceptible breathing and the beating of her heart. There she lay for hours, until at last she began to stir. Bleckwenn watched her, wondering whether her tenseness would return. Suddenly, the woman opened her eyes, looked at Bleckwenn, and said: "Doctor, what's the score?"

"Score of what?" asked Bleckwenn.

"Of the football game—Purdue-Wisconsin," the woman said. "They're playing it right now. You know that, Doctor. Who's ahead?"

This staggered Bleckwenn. He had been talking about the game while they were getting the woman ready for the amytal injection that morning. Clearly, her mind had been registering the events, although outwardly she was comatose and presumably insane. But now, lucid and out of her deep amytal anesthesia, this lady sat up, ate a hearty meal unaided, went to the bathroom under her own direction and smoked a cigarette.

As an unusual experiment in medical history, for the next two years this demented woman would wake daily out of deep sleep brought on by amytal and stayed clearheaded and sane for eight hours a day, every day. During that time, she would talk happily with her old father and mother, who were in tears to see her so much better. For seven to eight hours a day, she was sane, behaving in every way like a normal human being. Then, daily, she fell into a normal sleep. When she awoke, she was rigid and demented. After two years of this eerie routine, she died.

FOLLOWING THIS INITIAL "SUCCESS," Lorenz and Bleckwenn turned to others of the insane, those who were rigid, mute and so out of touch that they had to be tube-fed. Daily, the patients sat up like ladies and gentlemen to eat their dinner, after awakening out of deep sleep brought on routinely by amytal. After polite post-dinner conversation, they retired to a natural sleep. They woke the next morning— crazy, one and all.

In any large practical sense, the experiments were a failure. Lorenz could hardly advocate amytalizing the world's chronically insane to bring them out of it to be sane for eight hours a day.

But the question remained: what did this barbiturate, amytal, do inside the brain cells to remove the chemical block, the stymie that kept them from revealing the sanity deep in them, that had been there all along, that had never left them? Lorenz had no answer. But he knew one thing: when the answer came, it would be chemical.

Yet Lorenz was nothing if not a fair-minded man. Here were insane people whom he could make sane for eight hours. They gave him a chance to test the prevailing, popular psychiatric theory that severe insanities of unknown cause are NOT chemical but psychogenic. In other words, not chemical but only in the mind.

So Lorenz and Bleckwenn spent hours with these strange patients who had been utterly inaccessible. The conversational give-and-take that resulted was satisfying and hopeful. The patients told the doctors about their past lives. *Had they been thwarted?* Definitely. *Had they experienced frustrations?* Certainly. Understanding their past mental and emotional problems, Lorenz methodically tried to reason them away. The patients showed insight. They agreed they'd been foolish to feel frustrated. They were baffled that they'd had to withdraw into private worlds. Under this conversational guidance, they seemed happy. But that evening they fell into their natural sleep. And the next morning they woke up, demented.

During this time, Lorenz had only this shred of hope: these eight-hour lucid periods showed beyond a doubt that many desperate mental illnesses are chemically reversible. Yet the lucid periods were only intervals; the hopeful chemical reversibility of these insanities couldn't be made to stick; the mental illness remained—incurable.

There was a bright side though, not for Lorenz but for those poor devils, the patients. In their lucid intervals, they were happy that they were no longer crazy; and once insane again, they forgot they had been lucid. The dark side was for Lorenz. Buried under a sick brain's disordered action, he had discovered sanity. It was as if he were a scientific Moses forbidden his promised land.

THESE DAYS OF THE MIDDLE 1930s might one day be known as the time when new medical miracles were born in the field of mental health. While Bill Lorenz was on his search for understanding, halfway across the globe in Germany, Manfred Sakel of Vienna and Berlin, was working on his own cure for people deemed hopelessly demented.

Like Lorenz, Sakel never set out looking for a big cure. At the start, his modest aim was the cooling down of drug addicts wildly agitated when they were taken off morphine. He theorized about what goes on chemically in addicts' brain cells when they are deprived of opiates. His theory required that he test the effect of lowering the glucose in the brain cells of the unfortunate wretches.

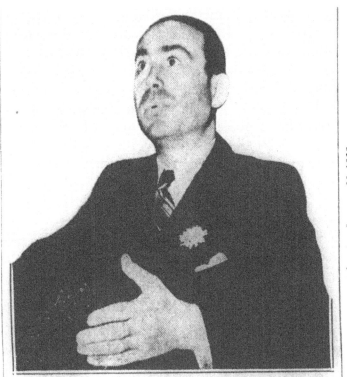

Dr. Manfred Sakel of the University of Vienna, explains to a group of American physicians how he discovered that insulin, life-saving diabetes remedy, can be used to shock hopelessly insane persons back to sanity.

So he began giving them, cautiously, shots of insulin. Then one day, one of these pitiful people—after an injection of the powerful diabetic remedy—began thrashing about in the convulsions of grave insulin shock and then drifted into a deep insulin coma. Sakel saved him with a quick shot of glucose.

However, as the patient came back to consciousness, he was utterly changed—calm, quiet, sane.

It was no happenstance. Deep insulin shock again and again wiped out the wildness of addicts deprived of morphine. But

Sakel was playing on death's doorstep. Driving his patients into deeper and deeper insulin shock in order to achieve his cure, he deprived their brain cells more and more completely of sugar. Of all the cells in the human body, the cells of the brain are the most delicate in that they cannot stand a starvation of sugar, their one food, for more than a few minutes. Glucose is the one fuel for the fire of life, and insulin, burning up that fuel, gives oxygen no sugar to oxidize.

Manfred Sakel noted that the terrible ordeal of the insulin shock did more than calm these agitated addicts. In some of them, it brought about a deep character change—for the better. If bringing a morphine addict close to death with insulin shock might do good for that addict, Sakel thought, why not try it on victims of dementia praecox, now called schizophrenia?

For Manfred Sakel, it seemed logical. The lunacy of a hopeless dementia praecox victim is a desperate thing, and doesn't that suggest desperate chemical measures for sick brain cells? And doesn't acute hunger brought on by insulin shock turn the insides of brain cells into a topsy-turvy turmoil? Mightn't it burn the sick old chemistry totally out of them, making way for a new, clean chemical kind of housekeeping?

It might if you didn't kill the brain cells while cleaning them. Such was Sakel's strange science.

In Germany prior to World War II, it would have been considered murder to lose a patient you had deliberately thrown into insulin shock. So now, night and day, Sakel was never without a hundred dollars in cash and his passport—with which to skip the country if the need arose. He began shocking assorted human beings—lunatics of unknown cause—with more and more insulin. He shocked them into the deepest possible convulsions and comas compatible with life.

By design and of set purpose, he did what every other physician in the world would at all costs have avoided.

So Manfred Sakel was, in essence, stretching out Bill Lorenz's lucid interval with bigger and bigger shots of insulin given daily. However, it wasn't like treating diabetes with measured units of insulin. There was no established "shocking" dose of insulin. He just had to feel his way, never knowing from patient to patient what would put them into shock. Sakel simply injected his insulin and hoped for the best.

In a rare case, one of Sakel's patients would go into a shock so deep that neither sugar nor adrenaline would bring him out. It was a shock from which there was no return. That or the patient would come out of such a shock a totally mindless vegetable or—even more rarely—the victim struggled out of this dangerously ungovernable shock as a new human being.

In the latter cases, it was not like the short lucid intervals that had so long tantalized Bill Lorenz. Instead, it was as if the patient's personality was reborn, and would likely remain so.

But for the majority of Sakel's patients, their return to the real world was not that spectacular. It was a long grind of insulin shocks daily, over weeks, even months. It was interesting how—in many patients but not all—each daily treatment seemed to wipe away another layer of insanity.

Early in the series of insulin shock treatments (as in Lorenz's lucid interval), there was a minute or two of sane talk amidst incoherent babbling. This lucidity was likely to come on a couple of hours after the insulin injection, just as the patient began to drowse toward the coma and possible convulsions. Sakel watched these moments of sanity lengthen, bit by bit, day after day, as he brought his lunatics into their insulin convulsions and coma.

For Sakel, it was like he was presiding over a battle—the sane self was fighting to throw out the crazy self a little bit at a time every day. Sakel saw unusual conduct in some patients during their last insulin shocks, when they were almost ready to be discharged from the hospital as "normal." As they drowsed off into their shocks, there was sometimes a last episode of craziness. Perhaps that devil of insanity was protesting being kicked out.

Manfred Sakel was surely one of the most daring men in the history of medicine. No insulin shock treatment could be called routine. He had to learn by experiment, he had to be quick, if convulsive death threatened, with an injection of adrenaline.

Sakel said, coolly, that he got his best results *as he approached the danger zone*. He pointed out that if physicians worried too much about danger, they'd forget the treatment's purpose.

This purpose was to try to rid sufferers of this mysterious affliction of madness.

IN THE MODERN TIMES OF 1956, the outcome of Manfred Sakel's tough, brave battle against mental illness has not been too happy. I remember writing about Sakel's strange adventures on death's doorstep and quoting published clinical evidence that stated how insulin shock treatment, if it was started within the first six months of serious mental sickness, could "cure" 70 out of every 100 patients.

Puzzled by this, one day I put a question to Jack Ferguson: if those figures were correct, shouldn't the population of the country's mental institutions have begun to go down, markedly, many years ago? That is, if insulin shock treatment was safe enough to be used routinely.

"Insulin shock isn't safe enough to be used routinely," said Ferguson. "And the mentally ill are not often admitted into state hospitals within the first six months of their serious sickness. And even when insulin shock is given to early, seemingly favorable cases, with what seems a fine result—the relapse rate is too high."

"But what about electro-shock?" I asked Ferguson. "That's safer than insulin, so they say."

"I don't use it in my service—the patients are too scared of it," he said.

It is an axiom of medicine that the earlier any illness can be treated, the higher the chances of cure. Why then was he testing his new chemicals, plus tender loving care, on the longest, most desperate insane? In this, Jack Ferguson seemed to me to be a tougher man than Manfred Sakel.

WHAT IS INSANITY?

When I say that Jack Ferguson is tough, it is only in the sense that he is tough on himself, not others. That's how he seems today, anyway, especially when it comes to the treatment of his patients, something that was not always the case.

An example is electro-shock therapy. We talked about the procedure at great length. Ferguson himself admitted to having used the procedure and found it effective in some cases.

"Then why have you given it up entirely?" I asked him.

"How would you like to prescribe that for poor devils who get under their bed and pull themselves up, holding on to the springs, hiding, the day they know they're going to get it?"

"But electro-shock has done a lot of good," I protested. "It's even kept early psychotics out of institutions."

"Yes, but they're *frightened* of it," said Ferguson. "It must do something bad to them inside their heads. I quit it the moment I knew the new neurochemical medicines were better."

When I say Jack Ferguson is tough on himself, it's only because he deliberately takes only the most regressed, difficult mental cases. He prefers to work with the so-called hopeless for the simple reason that he does not want to fool himself. He wants to be surer than sure of what he hopes to offer as a remedy. He wants to observe the healing effect of a remedy on those beyond hope, those people who are farthest gone.

Ferguson believes if a remedy cures the far-advanced cases, then he can be confident of its action on the earlier, milder ones. He didn't want to stir up false hopes among family doctors who might want to try his treatment on mental patients to prevent institutionalization. Ferguson didn't want to give false hope to people charged with caring for mentally ill spouses and children, families who might hear how his treatment helped release chronic, severely insane patients out of the asylum.

FERGUSON'S EXPERIMENTING LIFE is tough on him for another reason. The main mental illnesses of unknown cause—schizophrenias, paranoias, melancholias—differ sharply from physical illnesses such as pernicious anemia or bacterial endocarditis or cancer or the various diseases of the heart. All these have definite physical signs defined by concrete symptoms and laboratory tests. These tests tell you exactly what you are fighting and whether or not you are winning. But to diagnose the insanities of unknown causes, all Ferguson and his fellow psychiatrists have to go on is a kaleidoscopic, shifting sand of symptoms.

"Look, Jack," I recall asking him once. "You say there's a lot more to mental illness than this abnormal behavior you're treating here. But what's that 'lot more' you're always hinting at?"

"Well now, let's look at it this way," he began. Then he stopped, lost for an answer.

"What *is* mental illness?" I prodded further. "If all you experts have to go on is a mixed bag of symptoms, then aren't we all insane at times?"

"What do you mean?" asked Ferguson.

I told him then what had bothered me about myself for many years. It was a worry about my own mental condition, which I considered never too stable. I confided in Ferguson that I, too, have experienced a few of the major symptoms of the insanities of unknown cause:

Hebephrenia. The hebephrenic indulges in silly, senseless laughter. I've giggled uncontrollably many times.

Catatonia. The catatonic sits mute, rigid, speechless, dead-pan, as if in a deep pout. I've experienced this, too, and worried about it after coming out of it.

Paranoia. The paranoid has the delusion the world is against him. How often haven't I suspected darkly that somebody's out to get me? The paranoid has delusions of grandeur. How often haven't I felt the world was my oyster in my own field—only to fall flat on my face shortly after that?

Melancholia. The melancholic for no known cause is inconsolable. I've spent a few hours looking through dark-colored glasses at a world that turned out not to be so bad after all.

Mania. Manics dash about, wasting energy out of all proportion to the importance of their objectives. All my friends have seen me in bursts of such senseless activity, calling me, politely, a hypomanic—that is, a manic at large, not yet in a padded cell.

Hallucinative. Hallucinates hear bells or see little leprechauns walking in military order across the foot of the bed. In crowds, I've heard my name called by people who weren't there and spotted friends who were nowhere near.

"If these symptoms are what make up insanity," I said, "then I've been insane repeatedly. So what's the difference between me and your caged-up psychotics?"

"The only difference," he said, "is my patients make a career of it."

"But what's the cause of *their* making a lifework of those symptoms?" I prodded him. "And why do such symptoms bother *us* just for a little while and then fade away? Is insanity caused by a virus or viruses? What's the biology behind insanity? What's the chemistry of it? Do you know?"

"No, I don't know," said Ferguson.

"Does anybody know?"

"Nobody knows. Nobody I know of," he admitted.

"Then what's all this business of there being a lot more to mental illness than this abnormal behavior you're trying to treat here?" I asked.

Ferguson had no answer.

Among the main insanities of unknown cause—schizophrenia, paranoia, melancholia—there may be a few definite "diseases" that will, someday, be sharply defined chemically. Or there may be a dozen or a hundred. But how can you effectively fight them when you can't pin even one of them down?

Such is the toughness of combating insanity, the crux of Ferguson's experimenting life.

IN THE FICKLE WORLD OF MENTAL ILLNESS, there is a state of affairs that is still more strange—those cases where the cause of the mental illness is well known. These account for nearly half of all cases, according to Ferguson.

Ferguson proceeded to give me an impressive list of them. There was general paresis, due to the spirochete of syphilis;

this used to account for 30 percent of the male admissions to the hospital before the advent of penicillin. And Dr. Walter L. Bruetsch, of Indianapolis, has found that between four and five percent of patients in his mental institution also have rheumatic heart disease; a strange rheumatism that effects the brain and has made them demented. Deficiency of the B vitamin used to account for many admissions to mental hospitals in the South, before Dr. Tom D. Spies and his associates showed how vitamin B could wipe out pellagra. And there are chemical insanities caused by poisoning with metals such as lead, arsenic, and mercury—all of which may subtly bring on chronic mental illness. Opiates and cocaine and bromides, and even some antihistamines, can drive people mad. Tumors—meningiomas involving the frontal lobes of the brain—frequently begin by showing only mental symptoms. And simply being kicked by a horse or hit by a truck may leave brain injuries that addle their victims for life.

"That's real progress," I said. "Knowing the cause, you can prevent—even cure—that kind of mental illness."

"Yes, we can," said Ferguson. "But here's the catch: a lot of these organic mental diseases come to us with symptoms mimicking schizophrenias. So they often fool us."

I laughed. "So this is your psychiatric science," I said. "When you don't find a definite cause for somebody being crazy, you can just call it schizophrenia."

"Schizophrenia," Ferguson said, "isn't a disease or even diseases—it's a wastebasket for assorted mental symptoms."

"What a loony science," I said.

But Ferguson was not to be discouraged.

"Definite organic injuries and poisonings cause mental symptoms, and the symptoms of schizophrenia are the same. We'll find their cause, too, one of these days, don't you worry."

JACK FERGUSON HIMSELF, outwardly, is certainly no man to worry about these confusions in the not-quite-science of insanities. To illustrate his belief that you can cure someone without knowing what is specifically wrong with them, he proudly showed me one of his prize patients, a woman who had been confined to the Traverse City State Hospital for 51 years. For 30 of those years, her behavior deteriorated. Ripping her clothes off continually, she had been locked in a "specialing" room (hospital vernacular for seclusion). She lay on the floor, tense, mute, naked—less than an animal.

And now here she sat, a nice, old lady, past 70, who conversed a little, quietly and pleasantly. (You'll hear more about her later on in the story.)

"Please get that bogey word, schizophrenia, out of your head," Ferguson urged me kindly. "Don't worry about it." Then he gave me a capsule psychiatric sermon.

"Patients aren't diagnosed as schizophrenic until their abnormal behavior brings about their examination by learned authorities," said Ferguson. "And because these authorities don't know the cause of this abnormal behavior, they've built up a grand classification of various kinds of schizophrenia, based on various symptoms.

"Since it's difficult for any two learned authorities to arrive at the same diagnosis of the type of schizophrenia affecting a given patient—it's really just something to laugh at."

Ferguson's indifference to schizophrenia disturbed me. How could such an important, widely used, learned word be so preposterous, so misleading? I'd read earnestly with my own special Dutch perseverance in many big books about schizophrenia, and I found that Ferguson wasn't alone in his contempt of the mumbo jumbo connected with it.

"Schizophrenia is the great riddle of psychiatry," wrote Dr. Walter L. Bruetsch, who'd been Ferguson's teacher at Indiana University Medical School. Dr. Bruetsch pointed out how schizos can be every kind of crazy: they may be elated or withdrawn or expansive or regressed or aggressive or deluded or hallucinated or paranoid or melancholic. So—if the symptoms are interchangeable from patient to patient and from one day to the next—how can you separate, strictly, one type from another?

I brought this up to Ferguson, and he smiled at me benignly like the red-faced Hoosier Buddha that he sometimes seems to be.

"That's right," he said. "I've had patients who one day will laugh foolishly like a real hebephrenic and the next day will sit dumb and rigid like a catatonic."

TO TRY TO FIND ANSWERS, I dug into *The Biology of Mental Health and Disease.* It was a symposium on the last word in this field by 107 distinguished biologists, physiologists, experimental psychologists, brain surgeons, organic chemists and psychiatrists. Surely, here, I'd find facts about a warped body chemistry that set schizophrenics off from so-called mentally normal people.

In these papers, I found what seemed hopeful news about a chemical peculiarity of the adrenal glands of schizophrenics from Dr. Hudson Hoagland of Worcester, Massachusetts. The cortex, the outside layer or "bark" of the adrenal glands, secretes hormones that are the great normalizers of the organs of the human body, including the brain. When the human body is put under various physical stresses, the adrenal cortex sometimes hurries up to pour out extra hormones to help the body stand up to such emergencies. But when Dr. Hoagland put schizophrenics under such stresses, the adrenal glands of two-thirds of them failed to do their stuff. Their adrenals were underactive.

This seemed exciting. What, after all, when you came down to it, are schizophrenics? Dr. Hoagland says they're a group of human beings who have failed to meet the stresses of daily living and have then developed bizarre forms of behavior so that they have to be put into hospitals. Could it be that their brains got sick for lack of hormones from their adrenals?

Dr. Mark D. Altschule of Waverly, Massachusetts, also spoke at this symposium. Like Hoagland, he is a precise medical investigator. He had also studied the adrenals of schizophrenics, but contrary to Hoagland, he found their adrenals not to be underactive but *over*active.

To thrice confound the chemical confusion at this symposium, up rose Dr. Edwin F. Gildea of St. Louis. He reported that when he put schizophrenic patients under chemical stress tests, their adrenal glands acted no different from adrenals of folks who were sane.

So how could it be that three reputable, accurate, reliable observers and investigators all came up with different results for seemingly the same mental malady?

I wondered: could it be that each of the doctors was actually working with different kinds of schizophrenia? How could they know if they were testing the same condition?

WHAT IS INSANITY? The dictionary says the term is social and legal rather than medical, and it means a condition rendering patients unfit to enjoy liberty of action because of the unreliability of their behavior.

What are the psychoses, like schizophrenia, that make up the bulk of insanity? The medical dictionary says they're the deeper, more far-reaching and prolonged *behavior* disorders.

It was clear from the great symposium that, despite the devoted work of many intelligent men, their science is not yet sufficiently advanced to analyze what's at the bottom of abnormal activity. Though there's a lot more to mental illness than abnormal behavior, the trouble is that it is not known.

Jack's notion of mental illness is simply abnormal behavior, and his goal in treating it is just as simple—to coax the behavior of his pitiful sick people back to normal.

But, of course, we must ask: what *is* normal? The dictionary says it means being free from mental disorder, not insane or neurotic. To Ferguson it means something a bit more explicit. It means keeping your mental and emotional house clean, so that you can live fairly happily with yourself and others.

THROUGHOUT MY CONVERSATIONS with Ferguson, I kept thinking about my own mental state and the fine line of sanity. If I were asked to sum up my own mental and emotional life in a word, the word would be "turbulence." Friends call it energy, but they're wrong. Or if it is energy, it is not the good kind. It's impatience, inner agitation and tumult; it is constant inner unrest, tempestuousness. When it boiled up, my turbulence would hardly be called neurotic; it was not that feeble and mild. It was, underneath, one of the "deeper and far-reaching disorders." Psychotic. It expressed itself at its worst in a violent, ungovernable sensuality alternating with fiery, insatiable mental activity.

In the early 1930s, a real concern over my mental state forced me to the consulting room of a wise and sane psychiatrist, the late Dr. George Kirby of New York City. That kindly and understanding physician dragged out what gnawed inside me, the thing that made me so wild—at times to the verge of social irresponsibility. Dr. Kirby wrote it all down, while I wondered whether my confession would be used as evidence for a commitment. But, no. Although he had no pill for my turbulence, he helped me to begin to look into myself from the outside. He showed me that my one hope, the only possible medicine, was the love, the wisdom, the patience and devotion of my wife and partner, Rhea.

"How do you keep up with him—how do you stand him?" her friends were always asking her.

Only God knows how. But Rhea settled us away from the world, winter and summer, on the shores of Lake Michigan, and here by the lake's blue water for the past 24 years she has run what can only be called a one-patient institution. Here began what has been a long and slow and stormy recovery. Rhea—loving, lovable and lovely—guided it. Hard work in the woods with the crosscut saw and the double-bitted ax and long walks in the dunes and on the beach and the sting of Lake Michigan's cold surf—all these helped. Of course, the middle-aged cooling of the fires of energy also aided. The kindness of many scientific and medical friends—all better men than I—who believed in my work abetted my recovery. Getting to know that I couldn't be my own god, getting rid of my atheism, believing at last in God and learning to pray to Him—these medicines helped to fight the devil of turbulence. But the evil fires, though banked, still smoldered. Especially the mental "tempestuosity" and unrest. They were still there.

IN THE EARLY 1950s, my mental state along with what can

only be called a concatenation, led me inevitably to meet Jack Ferguson. It all began in line of my duty as a reporter, interested in the arrival in our country, from India, of the powdered root of a lovely shrub with bright green leaves and pinkish-white flowers. Its botanical name was *Rauwolfia serpentina*. But the people of India called it Pagal-Ka-Dawa. For hundreds of years it had been sold—across the counter, without any doctor's prescription—as a cure for insanity.

Utterly unscientific. Strictly folk medicine. But apparently not without a strange virtue.

For example, it is reported that Gandhi—by persistent chewing on this Rauwolfia root—gained the calm he needed to drive the British so wild that they went away, without a struggle, giving India back its independence.

In 1950, Dr. Robert W. Wilkins of Boston and Newburyport, Massachusetts, chanced to read an article by the Parsi physician Dr. Rustom Jal Vakil showing that this powdered Rauwolfia root was good for high blood pressure. Wilkins, though a brilliant and sophisticated clinical investigator, was not such a scientifically snobbish American as to scorn a tip from ancient India. In his clinic at the Evans Memorial Hospital in Boston, Bob Wilkins confirmed the solidity of this Parsi science, and that started a revolution in the treatment of deadly hypertension. It was the foundation of Wilkins' medical fame.

Besides helping other drugs curb dangerous high blood pressure, Wilkins discovered that Rauwolfia had another medical merit. It is characteristic of many hypertensive sufferers that they are inwardly turbulent. What Rauwolfia did to the quick-boiling emotions of certain of these patients amazed Harvard-taught, conservative observer, Wilkins. "The all-round improvement in some of my patients was so marked that what they said embarrassed me as their physician," he once told me. "They were lyrical about their sense of well-being on Rauwolfia drugs," he continued. (In modern medicine, lyrical is antithetical to scientific, and this naturally disturbed Wilkins. Rauwolfia couldn't be *that* wonderful.)

"What do those patients tell you, for example?" I asked.

"It's what they *don't* tell me," Bob said with a sigh. "Instead they tell me, I've never felt so well. . . . I haven't felt this good for years. . . . Nothing bothers me anymore because I just don't give a damn."

This supposedly happened so often and consistently—and faded so completely when he withdrew the Rauwolfia— that Bob had to believe them. And this happened not only to hypertensives, but to otherwise high-strung turbulent patients who did not have high-blood pressure.

Although this was outside his own scientific field, Bob Wilkins gathered up his professional courage. In a scientific publication, he wrote, "I have told many psychiatrists and others interested in psychotherapy that Rauwolfia is good psychotherapy in pill form." He had staked a second claim to his medical fame.

IT WAS WILKINS' WORK that brought me a step closer to meeting Jack Ferguson. The year was 1954, when Ferguson was helping to perform lobotomy operations on agitated psychotics at the Logansport State Hospital in Indiana. Ferguson loathed the severity of this terrible tranquilizing operation., and on a series of severely agitated crazy people, he decided to try Rauwolfia pills that had been left at the hospital by a pharmaceutical salesman.

To his amazement and delight, the pills worked as well as the ice pick. They even calmed some victims on whom the ice pick had failed.

At the same time period, my friend Dr. Frederick F. Yonkman, vice president in charge of research for Ciba Pharmaceutical Products in Summit, New Jersey, told me how Ciba's organic chemists had just crystallized a pure chemical out of the yellow powder of Rauwolfia. Fritz (aka Frederick) was excited. The crystals could be safely injected by vein or into the muscles of human beings. It seemed that these crystals were an anti-crazy quintessence. Although neither Fritz nor I had heard of Jack Ferguson, he told me how the new Rauwolfia crystals were knocking the turbulence out of certain violently insane patients, according to Drs. Robert H. Noce, David B. Williams, and Walter Rapaport at Modesto State Hospital in California. And this was confirmed by Dr. Nathan Kline at Rockland State Hospital in New York.

This pure Rauwolfia alkaloid was chemically labeled reserpine. It was already on the market with the trade name of Serpasil, said Fritz.

"The remarkable thing about Serpasil is that it tranquilizes turbulent people," explained Fritz. "But unlike a barbiturate such as phenobarbital, it doesn't turn them into zombies."

I myself had tried Serpasil. In 1954, I began taking it religiously, in what I thought to be a very small, completely safe dose—one-tenth of a milligram daily. The effect was a slow revolution.

For me it actually seemed like the beginning of the end of lifelong unrest. It was a damping down of the old impatience. Over the months came what Rhea and close friends called a character change. A slowing down of the old ferocious go-go-go. Internally, I felt the enemy—the turbulence—

fading away, changing into what Bob Wilkins's patients called the "don't-give-a-damn" feeling. And then after many months of sticking to that same very small 0.1 of a milligram daily dose of Serpasil, came a new feeling never experienced in my 65 years. Lethargy.

My lethargy began by edging close to what the Hindu mystics call nirvana. Yet, curiously, it wasn't in any way a zombie condition. It was simply not "giving a damn" about minor annoyances and frustrations. Then, this lethargy drifted into a mood that frightened me: though utterly rested and free from turbulence, I grew gloomy.

It was a Serpasil depression, a condition not typical of the small dose I was taking, but it was enough that I decided to go off the drug, only to find that—as the gloom and the lethargy and the don't-give-a-damn feeling and the wonderful tranquility vanished—my old turbulence reappeared.

So I went back on the same little Serpasil doses, and the events repeated themselves in the same sad cycle. My hope was blasted. It seemed I couldn't be tranquil, yet active. And at 65, I was haunted by the fear that my old turbulence—which at least had given me the big drive—was fading into the querulous, aimless restlessness of senility.

Then came help. It was a chemical called "analeptic." I heard about it from Fritz Yonkman, who said a fellow up at Traverse City State Hospital was using it successfully to boost physical and mental energy, "without giving patients the jitters."

That man was Dr. John T. Ferguson.

LOVE IS THE ANSWER

On Friday, March 9, 1956, Jack Ferguson spoke to an audience of 300 Michigan physicians who listened politely as he expressed his belief that admissions to mental hospitals could be cut in half if family doctors learned to use a combination of new medicines plus tender loving care to help their abnormally behaved patients. *Detroit Free Press* science writer Jean Pearson was also there, and wrote a front-page story with the Sunday morning headline, "Love Is His Answer: Doctor Tells How To Cure Mentally Ill," about Ferguson's work—along with a picture of his round smiling face.

"Last week," Pearson's article began, "Dr. John T. Ferguson gave one of his 1,000 women mental patients a twenty-three-cent gift. As she carefully cradled the small glass bowl with two goldfish, brightly colored shells and a sprig of greenery in her hands, the patient's face glowed."

"'Thank you, doctor,' she said softly.

"It was the first time she had spoken in fourteen years."

Like the recipe for Grandma's fudge cake, Ferguson's new treatment was so simple it was hard to explain and hard to duplicate on paper for others to follow. He fully admitted this to the room of doctors. In addition, Ferguson insisted that one add a pinch of understanding, a measure of kindness and a portion of love.

These ingredients took many shapes. For example, the small glass bowl. How did Ferguson sense that his gift would help to bring his patient out from behind her psychotic curtain? Where had Jack got his insight? In exactly what way did he learn the old and true lesson that kindness is a mighty medicine?

CAUGHT BETWEEN a Catholic father and a Methodist mother, Ferguson's boyhood in Indiana was not exactly easy. His father, a yardmaster on the Monon Railroad, was hell-bent on his son growing up to be a locomotive engineer. His mother dreamed that her boy might, instead, rise above his father's profession to become a doctor.

Like any normal child, Ferguson wanted his father and his mother to love him, so he grew up trying to appease them, simultaneously. But how can you fire engines on the Monon and study medicine at the same time? Ferguson gave no importance to this practical question. What fooled him into thinking he could do it was his feeling that anything he set out to do would be an easy task for him.

At age 11 he hired out in the summer as a wheelsman on a fishing tug on Lake Michigan out of Michigan City. He told the captain he didn't want any pay. Instead, he asked for all the discarded fish damaged in the gill nets, fish Ferguson would turn around and sell on a street corner on his way home. In this way he brought home many times the money they'd have paid him to steer the boat.

As a boy, Ferguson had not only sharp wits but savage drive. He decided his mother should love him more than his

youngest brother, who was somewhat frail, as well as being a
bed-wetter. To make his brother look even worse, Jack took
on two newspaper routes, morning and evening, and worked
in the drugstore after school. On top of this, he was doing
well in his lessons.

"I'd trample on anybody to get affection," Ferguson once
reminisced. "That was the first hint of a mad monster in me."

Unfortunately, his system of influencing his mother and
winning her affection worked in reverse. Graduating from
high school at 17, he left home. At the Gary, Indiana, steel
mills, he lied about his age—he was a big burly boy—and
wangled work as a common laborer, hoping to save money to
start premedical studies at Indiana University.

Starting out (this was 1925) at $4.40 a day, he worked ten-
hour days as a laborer, a chipper, an inspector, a cinder-snapper and a second helper in the slamming, banging heat of the
mills. By the end of the first year, he had worked his way up to
first helper, earning $14.00 for an eight-hour day.

In the tough environment of the mill, he learned to curse in
Polish, German, Spanish and Lithuanian. He learned to chew
snuff despite its nauseating effect on him. He trained himself
to swallow sandwiches—slabs of salami and hot yellow pep-
pers between two hunks of dark bread—without gagging or
filling his eyes with tears. He taught an illiterate Pole some
basic English, writing little words out in big block letters with
a piece of dolomite on the steel-mill floor. The men called
him "keet" (for kid) and liked him for the way he'd take the
dirty end of the stick on any job and kept smiling.

Ferguson had a way of fitting in. And yet his drive and a
sense of fate told him he was destined for greater things. The
mill with all his grimy-faced friends was just a means to an
end. So after a year and with some money in his pocket, he

finally bid them all a fond goodbye and enrolled as a premed major at Indiana University.

School proved a little more difficult and expensive than he expected. It would take Jack four years to complete his two years of study. His father couldn't see his way clear to help. but lost no time getting his boy a fireman's job on the Monon. Jack split his time between that and the university and finally, in 1929, he was set to enter medical school.

Marriage never entered Ferguson's young mind. If he had a plan at all, it was to *not* marry until he'd got his medical degree. But plans changed. He did marry and within a year there was a baby girl. To support his family, Ferguson took on extra hours on the railroad while trying to keep up a full medical course. He wasn't on the job long before he dislocated his knee and found he couldn't fire a locomotive with his leg in a cast. Weighing the options, he decided to drop out of school, his first year of medicine incomplete.

"I had lots of drive, more than anybody," Ferguson recalled, "but when I hit an obstacle, I tended not to bore in or get around it. I'd back away and try something else."

But the world again had other plans—namely the Great Depression. Ferguson went to work one day … to find he was out of a job. Now, with a wife, a daughter and a dream to be a doctor that seemed as far away as ever, he began to slip into depression.

Hopeless and suicidal, Ferguson contemplated his own death until the thoughts finally led to action. Numbing both his wrists with shots of Novocain, he found himself standing before a bathtub full of water where he cut down to the blood vessels of both wrists with a safety-razor blade. Ferguson did it this way, he recalled, out of consideration for those who would be called in later to clean up the mess.

IN HIS STORY TO ME, Ferguson was vague about what happened next. By his recollection, for the next ten years, he claims he became a scholar in the study of human frailty. After recovering from his injuries, he wandered into a series of constantly changing pursuits. He sold insurance, but the routine ultimately bored him until he lost the job. He was a bartender, where he learned a lot about alcoholic insanity. From there he used his college training to become a whiskey analyst for a distillery.

As a whiskey peddler, Ferguson's drive and his charm sent him on an energy surge similar to his days at the steel mill. He started selling booze in saloons and clubs; he sold whiskey to wholesalers; he got to know Ralph and Al Capone and quickly sold liquor in carload lots to his own distributors. He was a big operator, but secretly loathed it.

All the time medicine was calling him back. In the late 1930s, the chemical revolution was exploding, scattering its gifts of new sulfas, vitamins and hormones and promising new lifesaving power to the humble family doctor—that was what Jack had always wanted to be. He'd seen for years now alcohol's negative effect on human behavior—already there was scientific news from Dr. Tom D. Spies of vitamin extracts to reverse it. His smoldering passion for medicine flared into a flame.

So he told his wife he was quitting the whiskey business to try to get back into medical school. He had saved a bit of money, but far from enough. His wife, worried, asked pointed questions: *When would he be ready to support her? How long would it be before he got out into practice? Would the school want him, being away so long and after what he'd been doing?*

To me, in a masterpiece of brevity, Ferguson summed up what ultimately became the slow breakup of his family.

"There was some question of my ability to study, of finances for my family, et cetera," he said. "The result was my going back to school in 1941 at age 33, minus one wife and daughter."

THE MONSTER WITH

At Indiana University, a committee of medical professors didn't think much of Ferguson's rekindled ambition. To welcome him back, one of the professors handed him a lead pencil and asked him to retire to the next room to write them an essay describing that pencil. They gave him no credit for the courses he had completed a decade before and essentially told him he would have to start over.

Ferguson, however, would not be deterred.

Driven by the deep despair he felt in his own failings, Ferguson found a new determination to help the suffering. By this time, he was himself alone. His father was dead. His mother was in a nervous state and out of his reach. His wife and daughter had moved to California. But Ferguson used these troubles to his advantage.

With nobody around to distract him, he was alone with his ambition to become a doctor. He breezed through that premedical year the professors had made him repeat. After he had paid his tuition and laboratory fees for the first year of medical courses, his total capital was 98 cents, so he got a job tending bar from late afternoon till midnight after a full day in school. Many times, he studied most of the rest of the night to have the next day's assignments ready.

While tending bar, he met the cashier in the tavern—a girl named Mary. She was Italian. Her serious, sad face, hinting at a not-too-happy past, had a trick of a slow-breaking smile and her eyes were gray and lovely.

"When we first met, Jack was fat," she told me. "He weighed two-hundred-and-sixty-pounds and was so fat even the Army—which had a wartime need for medical students in the early 1940s—rejected him. He was so fat I wouldn't have anything to do with him."

To win Mary's heart, Ferguson recalls dieting down to 210 pounds and moving on the divorce from his first wife. He and Mary would be married in 1944.

In Mary's eyes, Ferguson went from someone she wouldn't look at to a man she found totally unique. At home, she worked while he studied—cooking, cleaning and spending many hours as a cashier to help keep him in medical school. For his part, Ferguson talked to his new wife as if she was an equal in his medical world.

"Jack was so kind and gentle. He was so patient about my ignorance," recalled Mary, adding that while she considered herself born on the wrong side of the intellectual tracks, Ferguson never made her feel that way.

Ferguson was studying at Indiana University in Bloomington in the early 1940s. Between work and school, he sometimes slept less than three hours per night, for weeks on end. Mary worried about his lack of sleep, combined with old "fits of restlessness" that began to reappear. Ferguson would sometimes fail to show up for dinner, only to phone her from somewhere—like Indianapolis—without explanation and saying only that he was sorry and was hurrying home on the next bus.

"When I would ask him why," said Mary, "he'd only reply that he was a damn fool and hang up. But he was so good-natured, always kind to me, so I didn't press further."

BY SPRING OF 1945, Ferguson was finishing the second half of his sophomore medical year, teaching and at the same time studying medicine. He was on fire and nothing could stop him. He was in the medical school at Indianapolis now, commuting on weekends to be with Mary in Bloomington as they couldn't find rooms in the wartime-crowded city.

Then, in May 1945, he was hit by a severe coronary heart attack. The doctors told Mary he was going to die, but after seven weeks in the hospital, he was discharged and brought home, where Mary nursed him back to health.

"The one comfort I found was Mary," Ferguson remembered. "Her love made me want to recover."

But while he was in the hospital, frightened he was going to die and fearful because he'd lost a whole semester of his sophomore medical year, Ferguson had found another comfort: barbiturates.

Following the heart attack, his doctors had given him barbiturates to calm him down and make him sleep. He took them in the hospital even when he didn't need them and then at home while convalescing.

"I knew it was wrong," he remembered, "but I still sneaked them. They blotted out my perspective of reality."

Ferguson's notion of reality was that his heart was going to conk out again and then he'd die or, at the least, be washed out of finishing up his M.D. The barbiturates took away the impeding sense of doom. But soon he was addicted to the little yellow capsules. In one instance, after a checkup at the hospital that showed his heart was doing fine, he and Mary were standing at the bus station, prepared to go back to Bloomington, and Ferguson felt the crowd pushing too close to him. He began to shake and—sure another heart attack was going to hit him but having no pills to calm himself down—he bolted from the platform and decided to hitchhike home with a driver who was clearly drunk.

Ferguson can't recall many of the details about the accident.

"I'll never forget the expression of the ambulance doctor when he helped lift me out of the wreck and wiped the blood off my face and recognized me," said Ferguson. Just an hour before, the same doctor who had seen him for the checkup was now treating him for a dislocated shoulder, a collarbone separation, three broken ribs and a five-inch gash on his forehead.

Who could blame Jack for pitying himself? In the hospital, again, he had time to rest and feel sorry for himself and sneak more and more of those little yellow capsules that made him forget reality. The little capsules were his friends. Meanwhile, Mary wangled an unfinished veterans' housing project shack so they could live in Indianapolis, and she landed a cashier's job at the University Medical Center to help keep them alive financially.

Ferguson's medical professors, who had initially dismissed him, proved surprisingly wonderful during his recovery. While he was missing a whole semester of his medical course, they gave him a job teaching surgical anatomy and put him in charge of the biochemistry laboratory. Ferguson had always had a chemical imagination. He could see the theoretical hexagons and pentagons and side chains of complex structural organic chemical formulas—three dimensional in space—as if they were real.

There was no doubt of Ferguson's great wits, but his behavior disturbed Mary more and more as he depended increasingly on barbiturates to get through the day.

"Up to this time," recounted Mary, "Jack had been gentle and kind to me. But he slowly began to get spells when he was real ugly. He would tell me to go away and express regret at ever marrying."

After such an outburst, Mary remembers her husband crying and telling her she was all he had in the world. Afterwards, he would work furiously. He started teaching surgical anatomy and biochemistry, his arm still in a sling after the accident. He mentally gulped down and digested great gobs of complex science, and it added to the turmoil of his brain, already overactive. He was frightened. All this chemistry that would give him a magician's power when he had his M.D.—what good would it do him if his heart conked again? So he took the little yellow capsules. Then he'd sleep a couple of hours and forget. As he gained more of a tolerance for the drug, it took more and more of them to kill the fear and calm him down.

DURING THOSE MEDICAL SCHOOL YEARS, this addiction was a secret between Ferguson and Mary. But he was on the verge of what the doctors kindly call a nervous breakdown.

"How did you keep your medical friends from knowing you were on barbiturates?" I asked Jack.

"I normally carried such a head of steam," he remembered, "that when I was underactive, on the capsules, I seemed to them to be normal."

On the whole, Ferguson and Mary's life was far from tragic. Dr. Harold E. Bowman, their closest friend in those days, remembers the Ferguson's place in Gravel Gulch as an open-house. Drop-ins were always made to feel welcome. The Fergusons were poor as a pair of church mice, but could always scrape up money for classmates who needed it. At parties, Jack had a taste for old scotch, bonded bourbon and imported gin.

Though now in his late thirties, there seemed to be no let up of Ferguson's drive; it was as if he was still in his teens at the steel mill in Gary. Besides making excellent progress in his regular medical studies and teaching biochemistry, Ferguson eked out a dime here and a dollar there preparing the cadavers for the students of anatomy. He got up early in the morning and hurried to do BMR determinations on patients in the hospital, or he brought oxygen to patients in need of it.

"Jack liked to take me along to watch him get those corpses ready for anatomy," remembered Mary. "He was so good to me the way he tried to teach me. He let me come with him to the pediatric wards. I was proud the way the kids loved him."

By 1946, Mary had given Ferguson the confidence to burn his bridges and give up 20 years of seniority as a fireman on the Monon and go for broke for his M.D. And in June of 1948, the goal he had been working and dreaming toward for 22 years was finally realized. At last, at age 40, John T. Ferguson was a certified M.D. He had done it.

THE DAY HE GOT HIS DIPLOMA, Ferguson was overjoyed and feeling that if he could only treat one patient on his own as a country doctor, he'd be satisfied. Only a year as an intern now stood between Ferguson and that dream.

"I was thankful and grateful to Mary for standing by me," recalled Jack. "But I was also hopped up with barbiturates."

Once, in a letter, Ferguson recounted to me what was going through his mind in those days:

"*In my last medical school years, I had lost the Ferguson that wanted to be a country doctor, that wanted to treat people as well as their diseases," he wrote. "I was the product of self-generated false ideas of grandeur. I was* THE *doctor. I was above the multitude. . . . They could come to me. To keep up this front, each time my conscience slipped through I'd take barbiturates until my conscience could no longer be heard. Though still vitally interested in the human side of medicine, money and power were now my guiding lights.*"

This was how he looks back on that crucial time. But his immediate problems were real enough. One night, while foggy from the capsules, Ferguson took a nasty tumble on his way to the bathroom and ripped loose his collar bone. Reluctant to call a doctor, and with Mary gone away on a trip, Ferguson took more barbiturates to kill the pain. He followed this up with codeine, six grains in all, and the next morning, he was higher than a kite when he made it to the hospital. He conned a friend into getting him 20 more barbiturates, which lasted no time at all. And when he couldn't get more, he went crazy, literally.

He hallucinated at work, imagining that in the next room doctors were operating on Mary. He heard them say she was dying. Then came the paranoia. In the days that followed, he complained bitterly that the doctors (his friends) were neglecting his shoulder. This was followed by delusions that he was up in an airplane with Jack Benny and Dr. Richey, showing them the details of an elaborate system that would put Indianapolis under their control. He finally became homicidal, threatening to kill an intern assigned to watch him after his friends began to worry.

"They did all they could until I was too rough and noisy," Ferguson remembered. "I was rough, and one man alone didn't dare touch me. Even though I still had the separated shoulder."

Today doctors would diagnose his condition as "acute barbiturate withdrawal psychosis." After the incident with the intern, Ferguson's doctors took control and transferred him to the BB ward of the hospital. It was the bull pen, the snake pit. He heard an iron door slam behind him, locking him in. It was the hospital's locked ward for disturbed psychotics. Here he was no longer John T. Ferguson, M.D., proud of being a house officer in the teaching hospital of Indiana University School of Medicine. Here he was Ferg—unshaven, sullen, mean and dangerous among a ragtag bunch of bums and drunks, all of them more or less off the beam.

After two weeks the withdrawal symptoms subsided and Ferguson was clear as a bell. He was signed out of the bullpen, but patching up the relationships with his peers and colleagues wasn't easy. People looked at him differently now. Instead of a doctor, they treated Ferguson like a patient recovered from an acute illness. Even so, they allowed him to return to work as an intern under the condition he stay dried out.

Fortified by remorse of how he treated the people around him—especially Mary, whom he had also threatened to kill before sending her away—Ferguson returned to work. But, secretly, he craved the pills. He eventually succumbed to the temptation, but resolved to be more careful, more clever about it this time. After all, he knew how to sneak the barbiturates without anybody knowing. He knew how to dose himself without the doctors suspecting. He could outsmart both the doctors and the barbiturates. He had a deep personal secret and was proud of it—he had so much more drive than ordinary people that he could dose himself delicately to keep his wild, overactive behavior down to what seemed normal—so long as he didn't take too many of the capsules.

JOHN FERGUSON GRADUATED and, while still "shaky," by his recollection, moved to Hamlet, Indiana—population 500—to set up his country doctor practice. In a town starved for medical care, Ferguson was an immediate success that summer of 1949. The citizens of Hamlet and its surrounding farm country started to raise $5,000 to equip an office for him, but they liked Jack so much that they raised $12,000—to be paid with interest at six percent—and they built him an office and bought him an automobile.

The new Dr. Ferguson did not have to wait for patients; from the start they had to wait for him, and why not? He was dry behind the ears; he was 41 years old. He radiated personality. He'd fought his way up from a steelworker, a bartender and a fireman on the Monon, teaching medical science and taking all of 20 years to earn his way through medicine. He seemed to know life and to know people as well as what ailed them. And his smile, let alone his medicines, made them feel they were going to be okay. From the start, his practice was swamped.

The Fergusons, as a couple, proved a great addition to the community. Mary became Ferguson's receptionist, his office janitor, his bookkeeper and she was keen as his nurse in emergencies, as well as his cook and housekeeper.

FERGUSON REMEMBERED that first year in practice as many days of long work and hardly any sleep. He loved it. As his reputation grew, the office in Hamlet became like a country fair and people flocked there from 20, 40 and 50 miles away, as if Ferguson were some kind of healer.

Ferguson seemed destined for the big time medically, but he showed Hamlet's citizens he was there to stay. He'd used the money they'd loaned him, not only to build his office, but part of it as down payment on the most modern X-ray and lab equipment and the most up-to-date antibiotics and other pharmaceuticals. To give Hamlet the best in medical science, Dr. Ferguson had gone in the hole about $50,000, or so it was rumored. Nothing was too good for Hamlet. And the people of Hamlet responded by showering him with gifts—from the fresh summer vegetables left by grateful patients to the autumn choice cuts of meat from surrounding farms.

"Jack was never one for sleeping, but the first sign Jack was back on barbiturates," recalls Mary, "was his speech."

The patients began to notice the kindly country doctor occasionally had trouble with his words. Nobody thought Dr. Ferguson was drinking—maybe it was that he never seemed to sleep. The good doctor never said no to anyone.

"Not saying no was my downfall," Jack claimed. "I fretted and worried and took pills and capsules only to need more pills to sleep. Then to run away from this foolishness, I took other pills and capsules, more and more of them."

Looking for a reason of why he went back to the pills, Ferguson blamed the nature of the job, which he says conflicted with his reasons for getting involved in medicine in the first place. He wanted to help people. He felt as if he made too much money for what he was giving back.

Of course, he was saving some lives, but that was antibiotics, not him. His practice began to feel like too much of a production line—one of shots and pills for conditions where tender loving care may have done more good.

Ferguson wanted to help people, not merely make money, and he was making too much money. His conscience, he says, became too much for him—so he smothered it with barbiturates.

FINALLY, ONE SUMMER DAY, Ferguson found himself lying in bed in a hazy barbiturate daze. A patient who had come from miles away was begging to see him. Mary was answering the phone, lying, which she hated to do most of all. The phone kept ringing.

"Knock yourself out. Get away from it. To hell with it," the little yellow capsules told Ferguson. So on that day in July 1950, at the end of a year of roaring success as a country doctor, Ferguson was finally carried out of his practice and into a locked ward of the Veterans Administration Hospital at Indianapolis.

During the next 13 months—from July 1950 to August 1951—Dr. Jack Ferguson was hospitalized three times as a barbiturate psychotic. Each time he heard the iron door of the locked ward slam behind him; each time it took longer for Dr. Bernard Frazin and his staff to dry Jack out of the poison of the capsules. Each time it took him longer to bounce back to normal and get back to his practice. Dr. Frazin begged him to stay in the hospital so he could find out, by psychotherapy, what was wrong with him. But Ferguson always talked his way out, promising he'd whip the problem every time.

Dr. Frazin, a kindly man with insight, advised Jack to sell his practice and get a job "in a more sheltered environment." Yes, in one of these loony bins, thought Jack. Never. He'd started out to be a great country doctor; he'd show them yet.

Mary was proud when Jack began again with a rush. If there were such a title, the big medical association might have elected him the best rookie country doctor of the year.

But one night, he was called to go out to a sick patient far away in the country. Yes, he'd be out in half an hour, mumbled Jack, thick-voiced. He fumbled into a new suit of clothes, stumbled out to his car, opened the door and fell down in the mud.

Mary desperately tried to make him get up, tried to lift him—no go. She had to get two neighbors to carry Jack back into the house.

"I was so humiliated," Mary reminisced, "but the Hamlet people were wonderful. They loved Jack and knew he was sick and forgave him everything."

Ferguson repaid the kindness of the citizens by suspecting they had it in for him. He no longer blamed himself for his tiredness; he no longer blamed his fits of depression on the barbiturates; he no longer blamed his manic spells on the coffee and caffeine he took to try to drive away the blues brought on by the capsules. He blamed Mary. She was the cause of all his trouble, he was sure. One night he drove her out of the house. She was ashamed to go to the neighbors. She stayed all night in the car in her nightgown and coat. Then, the next day, crying, he asked her to forgive him. He actually quit the capsules and got back to work. Then he decided to kill her.

"You have felt Mary's devotion, her humbleness through all this," Ferguson recalled, trying to explain it to me. "I thanked her by loading *her* up on barbiturates … more and more. When she was dying, I came to and, for the first time in months, I was a doctor."

Ferguson's method of snapping himself out of his psychosis was a bit rough on Mary, but for a moment he was a doctor again, giving her stimulants and intravenous injections, feeding her and nursing her and saving her life. But his clear-headedness only lasted till Mary recovered.

Then his twinges of remorse—Ferguson's term for his blues—drove him back on the capsules. He developed hallucinations—D.T.s in Technicolor, he called them. He fell on the floor and Mary couldn't get him into bed. Everything was like a kaleidoscope. He'd move his head and there'd be a new picture. Then the brightly colored designs were covered with hairs. He staggered to his feet, but the room was full of chairs and he couldn't get out of it. He called for Mary, but he couldn't get to her; her voice came from far away. She got him to bed, but every time he closed his eyes there were those whirling colors.

Ferguson remembers taking enough barbiturate to snow him under for two days, but he couldn't seem to die. There wasn't enough barbiturate in the world to kill him. He flubbed his suicide—just as he'd fizzled out as a country doctor.

ON DECEMBER 1, 1951, John T. Ferguson, M.D., left his practice in Hamlet. He simply locked his office and house and went away. He dried himself out just enough to get a job in the Veterans Administration Hospital in Marion, Indiana, and within two weeks he was fired when they found him sneaking barbiturates. Ferguson was again returned to the locked ward of the V.A. Hospital. Through it all, Mary stuck with him. She was all he had.

This time, however, when Ferguson dried out from the barbiturates, his personality failed to bounce back. In group therapy sessions, he found himself bursting into tears when anyone so much as looked at him. He could give his old doctor, Dr. Frazin, no reason for his sadness. The staff believed Ferguson to be a good candidate for electro-shock, but Dr. Frazin opposed it. He told his associates that if he were psychotic himself, he'd not want that kind of treatment. Dr. Frazin was a kind man, and dimly this came through to Ferguson—here was a doctor who wouldn't hurt him. Now he began to react to a strange new medicine.

There was an attendant named Griff and another husky attendant named Terry who treated him like a human being, not a crazy hop-head, when they helped him to bathe and dress. It was tender loving care. Let's condense it to a four-letter word: it was *love,* this new medicine.

WHAT IS THIS MYSTERIOUS MEDICINE? I scanned a medical dictionary and came to the word "lovage." This is defined as the root of an umbelliferous plant, the extract of which is supposed to stimulate menstruation and also relieve flatulence, but the word *love* is not found in Dorland's medical dictionary.

Dr. Frazin suggested to Ferguson that it might help his deep blues if he'd talk over his past with a sympathetic psychiatrist. During his first three visits to the locked ward, Jack had turned down this advice. "But this time I was cornered," he admitted, "I had walked out on my practice. I had gotten canned. I had nothing but Mary, and she just about had her fill of my abnormal behavior. There was no way to go but up, I couldn't sink any lower."

Through Dr. Frazin's kindness, Dr. Elwood Phipps and, later, Dr. Palmer Gallup, became Ferguson's professors in a one-man institute of the higher study of psychiatry—it made his first experience in the bullpen during his internship seem like a kindergarten.

Dr. Phipps and Dr. Gallup didn't tell Ferguson how badly he had behaved in the past nor how to behave in the future. Instead, they asked him to try to write memos on what he thought had been bothering him. "I found," Ferguson said, " if something bothered me, if I wrote it down, the trouble dissolved for a time," he said.

During sessions, Dr. Gallup would then read Ferguson's memos back to him. But instead of scolding him for his deplorable behavior, Dr. Gallup would ask him to explain why he felt the way he did about things. In this manner, Ferguson says he began to understand his beastliness. After six months in the hospital, he had dug so far into his own dark depths that he began to see a changed picture of himself. No longer was he the self-made doctor with dynamic energy; no longer was he the smiling personality who could charm the birds out of the trees. From his boyhood, he had had his own secret goal: it was for himself. He'd trample anybody, he'd walk on the dearest, he'd stamp on Mary to reach this goal: the aggrandizement of Jack Ferguson.

LOBOTOMY DISCIPLE

I N MAY OF 1952, JACK FERGUSON started life over. He got himself a job as a resident psychiatrist at the state hospital in Logansport, Indiana, a position typically reserved for young residents looking to pass the specialty board examinations that would start them on careers in private practice.

The duties of a so-called "ward walker" are light. But Ferguson was not content to merely coast. No sooner had he arrived at Logansport Hospital than he began working into the night. He brushed up on neuroanatomy and dug into the intricate details of the topographical anatomy of the human head. He learned it inward, from the scalp through the skull into the secret depths of the human brain. Nights after his sad day's work as a ward-walking doctor, Ferguson practiced operations on the heads of patients who had died.

Nobody stopped him. There is always plenty of room at the bottom as well as the top. And now, alone, Ferguson began to study a strange new branch of psychiatric science. Night after night, he dug into the writings of a bold and brilliant neurologist, Dr. Walter Freeman, the American pioneer of psychosurgery, and was entranced by the romance of this new surgical discipline. These bone-drilling, brain-slashing operations had been developed by a Nobel laureate Portuguese with the

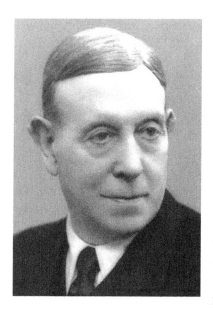

TWO EUROPEANS SHARE 1949 NOBEL PRIZE IN MEDICINE

Dr. Antonio Egas Moniz, Lisbon, Dr. W. R. Hess, Zurich, Get Award for Brain Research.

STOCKHOLM, Oct. 27 (AP)—The 1949 Nobel prize for medicine today was awarded to two European doctors for their study of and work with human and animal brains. They are:

Dr. Antonio Caetano Deabreau Freire Egas Moniz, 75 years old, one-time Foreign Minister of Portugal, honored for developing an operation to help persons suffering mental illnesses by severing some of the nerve connections of the brain. This operation, called a prefrontal lobotomy, has been helpful in treating schizophrenia (split personality) and paranoia (persecution mania).

strange name Egas Moniz. These Moniz operations had been made more practical and widely useful by Walter Freeman, who had simplified them to what Freeman called a "minor operation."

Ferguson was intrigued but wondered how he—a 44-year-old, ex-addict—could ever be clear-brained and steady-handed enough to start this so soon after fighting his way out of the stormy weather of his own psychosis? In fact, he was soon deep in a drive not only to learn, but to improve the ultramodern art of psychosurgery, all while shaking off his own mental illness under the guidance of Dr. Gallup.

There had been no shock treatments, no knives to cut out Ferguson's insanity. What was Dr. Gallup's elixir? What was it that so spectacularly transformed Ferguson from an unshaven, self-pitying, tear-stained, melancholic derelict into a surgical investigator on fire to try to heal the hopelessly insane?

I OFTEN ASKED FERGUSON what he thought the secret was to Dr. Gallup's treatment, and always he insisted it was Dr. Franzin and Dr. Phipps—and especially Dr. Gallup—who made him dig up and face the bad deeds he had done.

"I'd forgotten those bad things because they hurt me," he explained. "For me to remember them would have interfered with my believing what I liked to believe of myself."

Facing the bad in him, the "mad monster," seemed to clear up his thinking and clean out his brain. He fancied his years of stormy weather as having been a battle between Goliath and David. "In the Bible story," said Jack, "if David had not won, it could have been the end of mankind." Now he had faced that mad monster in himself.

"Who was your David?" I asked.

"The David was a weak little inner self in me."

"You mean, your conscience?"

"I suppose that's what we've got to call it," he admitted.

The thought was quaintly original, more poetic than scientific. Since there is no anatomical location for this mystery called "conscience," you could hardly expect Dorland's medical dictionary to define it—and it doesn't try to. But since this conscience was Jack's mighty medicine, I looked it up in *Webster's New Collegiate Dictionary*, which gives plain answers to ignorant people asking simple questions.

Conscience is the sense or consciousness of the moral goodness or the blameworthiness of one's own conduct, intentions, or character, together with a feeling of obligation to do right or be good.

In our inquiry into the mental and emotional factors that had brought about Ferguson's swift upsurge to a clear-headedness he had never felt before, this definition of conscience sounded a bit out of Sunday school, rather than a medical class. Discussing it with him, I groped for a somewhat less mealy-mouthed word than "conscience."

"Wasn't this rugged business of taking your life apart, looking at all of it and admitting and remembering and reminding yourself of all the bad—wasn't the big result of it your getting to be honest?"

"Exactly that," said Ferguson.

Then he gave me an example of this mighty medicine in action.

"It seems so easy and right to talk with you about myself," he said, "to pour out to you and Rhea the details of a crazy, mixed-up past. As I tell it, it makes me wonder how one man can get himself so all-screwed-up and live to tell it."

Honesty. This was Dr. Gallup's elixir.

FERGUSON HAD ALWAYS HAD GREAT WITS, and despite his total crack-up at Hamlet, he must have had a lot of them left to have been able to write his way out of his insanity under the guidance of Dr. Gallup. But then, don't great wits often go along with mental instability? John Dryden, who was only a poet, not a psychiatrist, thought so when he wrote more than 200 years ago:

Great wits are sure to madness near alli'd

And thin partitions do their bounds divide.

But considering his deep psychosis when he made his last grab for sanity, how did he have enough wits left for Dr. Franzin and Drs. Phipps and Gallup to reach him at all? How come he was still accessible to Dr. Gallup's psychotherapy? When he tried to explain it to me, he kept damning himself as a barbiturate bum. "I was limp and higher than a kite when I got to the V.A. hospital that last time," he remembered, "but not a total zombie, as most severe psychotics are when they get to mental hospitals."

From a source other than Ferguson, I found a possible clue to how he could be reached by Dr. Gallup's method, despite being diagnosed as crazy. It flashed over me during a study of *Psychosurgery* by Walter Freeman and James W. Watts. This amazing blend of the neurologic, psychiatric and surgical sciences explained how these disciplines are used to track down and scotch the invisible enemies of sanity that warp our brains. Dr. Freeman traces the deterioration of a schizoid personality, like Ferguson, into a schizophrenic lunatic, out of touch with reality. Reading this sad story, I reasoned that if Jack Ferguson had not become a barbiturate bum, *Dr. Gallup's psychotherapy might not have been able to help him at all.*

But what excited me most about Walter Freeman's story of how a schizoid personality may drift into downright madness—and the description fit Jack Ferguson like a glove—was the notion that a schizoid personality may often try to perfect himself for what he fancies will be his future greatness. The outer Ferguson was friendly and congenial, but the inside Freeman was schizoid to a T—struggling toward his ideal of the *perfect* country doctor; treating whole human beings, not their diseases; following his patients from cradle to the grave. This was his self-centered, ingrown thinking. This was his ambition, *his secret goal*, as he himself called it. Yet, as a model of the country doctor of his dreams, everybody must love him—his mother, his father, his first wife and daughter—and to bring that about he must please them all by becoming a locomotive engineer, a big whiskey businessman and a doctor all in one. Spreading himself too thin—for all his great wits and terrific drive—he failed, and that failure baffled Jack Ferguson.

In his book, Dr. Freeman explains what may then happen to such a self-centered, ingrown man: he strives for unattainable perfection. He magnifies his dreams of future glory. He becomes obsessed with these dreams only to turn in on himself and away from the world more and more. He becomes a ruminator, chewing the cud of his fancies and bringing them to mind, mulling over them again and again. Then they become fixed, become obsessions, overwhelming the machinery of his thinking, clogging the normal working of his brain. This was the embodiment of Ferguson when his coronary heart attack hit him in medical school. That disaster threatened to blast all hope of his ever becoming a country doctor.

"A normal individual when faced with such problems," wrote Walter Freeman, "may say to himself, 'to hell with it,' and go back to reading the comic strip." But the schizoid personality, unable to solve the problem, becomes more obsessed with it. And that is what I believe happened to Jack. When Ferguson couldn't rid himself of trying to imagine ahead into the inscrutable unknown of his future, he became more self-centered and scared. "Autistic [self-centered] thinking leads to fear," writes Freeman, "and fear is the most exhausting experience."

When Ferguson took his first tottering step toward becoming the sure-footed clinical investigator that he is today, his first science was not born from being rational, but instead from desperation. His crazy experiment smacked of Boss Kettering's definition of scientific research: "What're you going to do when you can't go on doing what you're doing now?"

After his accident and later, while leading his private practice, Ferguson often lay awake at night, worried and frightened and exhausted by his fear. Perversely, his tired brain grew more alert, seemingly as a result of its fatigue and insomnia. What was Jack going to do when he couldn't go on doing what he was doing now? He'd get to rest his overactive brain.

So this, I believe, lay at the root of why Ferguson began doping himself with the little yellow capsules. They tranquilized him, imperfectly, but enough to get him through his country practice in Hamlet.

In Hamlet, he was a perfectionist, not only in the quality of his medical work, but in the speed of his wanting to show the world he was going to be the perfect country doctor. He'd show the world in a year. Quickly he was making a barrel of money. Immediately his patients loved him. Yet he was failing. He knew he wasn't giving all his patients all the country doctor must give to be great. Ferguson felt like a phony, which conflicted with his inner battle for perfection.

In *Psychosurgery,* Walter Freeman tells how, when psychotics (like Ferguson) come under the care of psychiatrists, they've built up their inside, unreal world to a point where their early, self-centered thinking is lost in a welter of confusion, of hallucinations, of their not knowing what or where or how or when. They've been too hurt by the cruel indifference of the outside world to go back to it. They've been defeated too often, writes Freeman, in their attempt to visualize the future. They've run away into the secret world of their psychosis and they like it there, away from everybody, away from the very doctors who try to help them. "Patients in this state are relatively inaccessible to psychotherapy," says Walter Freeman.

But once in a locked ward, Ferguson, although crazy, was still in reach of the kindly questioning of Dr. Phipps. He was still accessible, which caused me to wonder: could the barbiturates have guarded him while they poisoned him? Did experimenting with barbiturates tranquilize him enough to leave the door open for Dr. Phipps and Dr. Gallup?

When Ferguson left the V.A. Hospital, it seemed that in the fire of that ordeal the old Ferguson had died, leaving a new version that was clearheaded and insightful. "I left the hospital to go into psychiatry," recalls Jack, "as I knew it was the only way to save my life."

It was his insight that he knew he would have to go on saving his life all the rest of his years. His medicine was strictly unmedical; it was in no sense chemical, it was only expiation. Yet it had a psychiatric precedent. Alcoholics Anonymous save themselves by expiation, by keeping on with the work of salvaging other alcoholic psychotics. "As others gave me a helping hand," he said, "I in turn must be only a servant." After his wonderful doctors and nurse attendants had saved him, Ferguson was compelled to help others. This new altruism reminded me of a quote by Ernest Renan:

To take action in the world, your own self must die.

In his new start in life at the state hospital in Logansport, Ferguson sought to right all his previous wrongs. The only obvious obstacle was that his new patients were seemingly

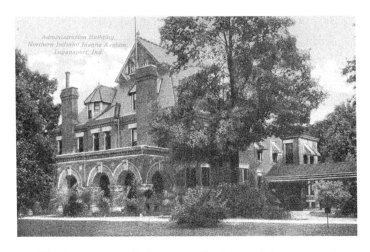

not like him. Instead, they were far beyond the point where psychotherapy and a reassuring talk could help.

"You could reassure them every day for months," said Jack, "and at the end of it they'd look at you, blank, and you were lucky to get 'glub' for an answer."

Still, believed Ferguson, all of them were human. All of them deserved a chance and his best effort to bring them back to reality. It was with this renewed purpose that he started helping neurosurgeon Dr. John A. Hetherington of Indianapolis, who was doing a few prefrontal lobotomies on the mentally sick at Logansport hospital.

FERGUSON REMEMBERED cramming himself on the psychosurgical writings of Walter Freeman whose expressed goal was to make his lobotomy so precise, so practical, so routine that it could be used to quiet the screaming bedlam of the disturbed wards of mental hospitals and send more and more hopeless patients home from them, sane.

The story is well known, but worthy of repeat. When Free-man approached the eminent psychiatrist Dr. William A. White for permission to try the new prefrontal lobotomy on the insane in the world-famous St. Elizabeth's Hospital in Washington, D.C., White refused. "It will be a hell of a long time before I let you have permission to operate on any of *my* patients," he roared. And that seemed that. But despite Dr. White's indignant thumbs-down, now there was a long waiting list of insane candidates for Freeman's lobotomy at this same St. Elizabeth's.

Freeman, back in 1936, had shown his faith in the then obscure Portuguese physician Egas Moniz. The hunch that had started Moniz on his stab-in-the-dark into demented people's brains was somewhat far-fetched and certainly strange. At a scientific congress in London in 1935, Egas Moniz had heard Professor John Fulton, Yale University physiologist, explain how he had experimentally mutilated the brains of certain trained chimpanzees. They had been very sad, and the operation—unintentionally—had made them happy. It was purely scientific. Professor Fulton was not crusading for happiness among chimpanzees. These sad apes were mean, difficult, depressed—neurotic— when they failed at their lessons. Professor Fulton, with his associate, Dr. Jacobsen, had cut the frontal lobes, the supposed highest seat of intelligence, out of their brains. Amazingly it did not turn the chimps into zombies.

"They acted," wrote Professor Fulton, "as though they'd joined the happiness cult of Elder Michaux and placed their burdens on the Lord."

It was uncanny, this operation. If the lobotomized apes failed at their lessons, they didn't worry. They weren't can-tankerous; they seemed not to give a damn. But they were

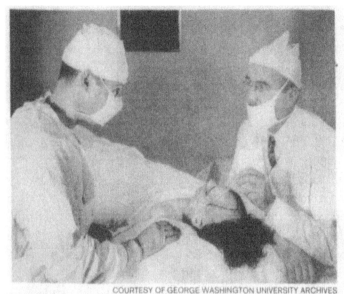

COURTESY OF GEORGE WASHINGTON UNIVERSITY ARCHIVES

Walter Jackson Freeman, right, operates on a lobotomy patient in 1942 with neurosurgeon James Watts.

still intelligent. They were apes with brand-new personalities, changed for the better. They were amusing laboratory curiosities.

But Walter Freeman reported how these happy apes didn't seem laboratory curiosities to Egas Moniz. They set him afire. Moniz hurried to seek out Professor Fulton, asking that distinguished scientist if it wouldn't be possible to apply his operation to human mental sufferers. Moniz compared the querulous, deluded, agitated, obsessed lunatics in asylums with these apes, happy and calm after the loss of the front of their brains.

But the Moniz project "was too much for Fulton," wrote Dr. Freeman. It was outside Professor Fulton's academic sphere. Also, Egas Moniz might be a bit overbold. When you cut out an important part of the brain you can't put it back. And though the proposed operation might make sad, crazy people happy, what would be their eventual fate?

READING FREEMAN'S STORY, Ferguson was initially excited by Moniz's faith in Professor Fulton's pure science and by Dr. Freeman's excitement at the first results of a handful of insane patients, operated upon by Dr. Almeida Lima and Dr. Egas Moniz in Lisbon, Portugal. These Portuguese pioneers had bored holes through both sides of the skulls of 20 insane patients. With an ingeniously devised knife—the leucotome—they cut the masses of nerve fibers that connected the frontal lobes with a mysterious spot in the middle of the brain—the thalamus. The frontal lobes are supposed to be for thinking and the thalamus is thought to be a powerhouse for emotions; and there is deep dispute—too deep for me— as to the significance of this frontal lobe-thalamus hookup. Anyway, after the nerves in the brain were cut, Moniz and Lima were happy to report that seven of their 20 demented patients recovered their sanity. Seven more were definitely improved … and none died.

But what excited Ferguson was the brilliant way Walter Freeman had carried on with these lobotomies from where his mentor, Moniz, left off. Freeman pointed out that since the lobotomy operation was not only effective but dangerous, it was of prime importance to follow up its results. He kept in constant touch with his operated patients and their families by mail. Patients also returned again and again for checkups and Freeman visited them in their homes from coast to coast. He was modestly proud of the ten-year follow-up of the first 20 mentally ill people he had lobotomized in 1936.

DOWN BROS. and MAYER & PHELPS, LTD.

LEUCOTOMY INSTRUMENTS

devised by

J. S. MacGregor and J. R. Crumbie

Vide LANCET: " An Improved Leucotome."—May 30, 1941.
Ibid.—" Surgical Treatment of Mental Diseases."—July 5, 1942.

Head Office : 92-94, Borough High Street, London, S.E.I
Showrooms : 32-34, New Cavendish Street, London, W.I   Welbeck 3764

Ten years later, there were fourteen survivors. Four were employed; four were keeping house; four were living at home; only two were confined to mental hospitals. And mind you, before the operation, shock and all other treatment had failed for these patients; there had been no hope for any of them; they would have been permanently disabled. Since 1936, Freeman and his co-worker, Dr. Watts, had slashed the brains of many hundreds of nervously broken and downright insane people. Result overall—75 percent could live at home, away from mental hospitals.

Ferguson studied reports by other neurosurgeons who had tried to confirm Walter Freeman's findings. From a U.S. Public Health Service survey giving the overall results of a total of 10,000 prefrontal lobotomies, there'd been good results in one-third; fair results in one-third; no response in the rest. And the operative death rate was only three percent.

Wasn't this real progress against mental illness, reasoned Ferguson, when practically all those stabs in the dark into the front of sick brains, by surgeons of different degrees of competence, had been risked for hopeless mental illness only?

THOUGH THEY HAD NEVER MET, Walter Freeman became Ferguson's teacher. What a tough man Freeman must be, he thought, as he read the histories of patients whose families had come to Freeman, pleading. In life, wrote Freeman, these patients—like Ferguson—had been failures harassed by doubts, fears, depression and suicidal ideas. Like Ferguson—who himself was a candidate for Freeman's operation—they'd been tormented by hallucinations.

One thing troubles Ferguson—the fact that those rescued by the procedure had to trade something precious for the relief of their mental anguish—the emotional component of the illness. "Abolishing emotions," wrote Dr. Freeman, "does away with certain concern for the future … as regards the individual himself.… The patient has enough foresight to carry out effective work but is definitely not concerned about personal failure, disease, death and damnation."

Amputating emotions also amputates initiative and the "brain power" for creative work. To this hazard, Walter Freeman noted only a couple of rare exceptions. The lobotomy had returned hundreds of mechanics, clerks and other routine workers to full employment, but it had never been shown to rehabilitate a doctor to his practice or a writer to his art or a scientific man to his research.

"Look what I've escaped, not having a lobotomy," recalled Ferguson. "And God knows I needed it."

Dr. Freeman would not perform the brain operation unless the patient was threatened by permanent disability or suicide, and then only when insulin or electro-shock treatments gave no promise of success. "Prefrontal lobotomy," wrote Freeman, "is the last resort, the end of the line."

For all of its salvage of the seriously insane, the standard prefrontal lobotomy had other drawbacks. Deep cuts into the front of the brain often relieved victims of years of terrible tension and sadness. But just as often, for some time after the operation, the newly "sane" patient might behave like a boisterous, mischievous, irresponsible child. It was uncanny to watch these people grow up out of this surgically induced childhood. But Freeman admitted no other disorder may last so long with so many problems of convalescence as recovery after prefrontal lobotomy.

Walter Freeman would take no candidates for lobotomy without their families realizing the rugged time they might have training their dear one to be a grownup again, even to housebreaking the patient literally as well as figuratively. Psychosurgery was no cure for insanity; it only opened the door to reality.

Could tender love care complete the recovery, reasoned Ferguson.

THE EARLY LOBOTOMY PROCEDURE was a lengthy one, so Freeman developed a new brain-slashing trick that took minutes instead of hours. He perfected an operation devised by Italian surgeon A. M. Fiamberti. Instead of laboriously boring holes in the skull, Freeman quickly and neatly slashed the sick brain with an ice pick driven up inside the skull through the bony roof of the sockets of the eyes.

This was the "transorbital lobotomy," done so quickly that Freeman called it a "minor operation." It was followed by no stormy childish convalescence. It was over in minutes before an observer thought it had barely begun. Why shouldn't psychosurgeons—with American production-line ingenuity—begin to empty mental hospitals?

During those early years at Logansport, Ferguson became a fiery disciple of Freeman's work. Boning up on his neuroanatomy so he could visualize the brain's inner topography with his eyes shut, Ferguson began his operations by feeling landmarks on the outside of the head. Verifying his book knowledge, he drove an ice pick up over the eyes, up through the roofs of the eye sockets of dead people and made sweeping slashes that were bolder and bolder in those dead brains. In this manner, Ferguson perfected a more drastic, more thorough transorbital lobotomy. Or so he hoped.

"The technique is as follows," wrote Jack in a memo to the superintendent of Logansport State Hospital and to its consulting neurosurgeon, Dr. Hetherington:

After the usual preparation, the lids of one eye are held open with an eye retractor. The point of the pick is placed against the orbital roof (top of the eye-socket) and while held parallel with the nose is driven in until the five-centimeter mark on the pick is opposite the upper eyelid—

Ferguson, the fledgling psychosurgeon, then specified in precise figures of so many centimeters the sweeping cuts of the pick inside the brain. Toward the inside, toward the outside, toward the top, toward the bottom of the front of the brain, the cutting guided by the pick hitting this and then that bony landmark outside the skull.

With the above described maneuvers we feel a maximum

transorbital lobotomy is done, thus giving results similar to the standard operation.

Hetherington was impressed and, later, collaborated with Ferguson (along with Dr. E. Rogers Smith, and Dr. John A. Lawson) in the latter's first scientific paper for *The Journal of the Indiana State Medical Association* in 1954.

Ferguson's modification of Walter Freeman's transorbital lobotomy could be completed in three minutes' time. While the standard prefrontal lobotomy carried a mortality of between two and three percent—low considering its power of bringing back sanity—the transorbital operation seemed far safer. In their last 162 lobotomies, Ferguson and his associates reported they had not had a single death.

At the time, there was a touch of the radical in Ferguson's feeling toward the grim and beautiful psychosurgical art. He did not try for good statistics. He did not choose "the most suitable cases." Walter Freeman had warned that deteriorated schizophrenics were unchanged by prefrontal lobotomy. But Ferguson tried his operation even on the most hopeless cases. He tried them all and found that while his new transorbital operation seemed to be standing up to Freeman's standard prefrontal lobotomy, and these mentally sick patients often behaved much better after the operation, the big cut in their brains left them lacking. "It was odd," explained Jack, "they couldn't seem to finesse; they couldn't plan ahead."

This seemed true of all the lobotomies, but there were exceptions that made Ferguson happy. For example, there was this case of the schizophrenic woman, age 39, who'd come to Logansport wildly paranoid and who had shown only slight, and then transitory improvement after 60 insulin shocks. After a lobotomy in March 1952, she appeared saner and was finally furloughed in August. Back for a checkup in June

1953, the lady was anxious for her final discharge papers. Her brother reported that his sister has made an excellent adjustment on his farm and was considered one of the most ardent workers on the premises.

FINALLY, THE DAY CAME when Ferguson would meet Dr. Walter Freeman at a neurological society meeting in Chicago. Ferguson remembered the preeminent doctor was very kind. "He was a tall man with a mustache and a little goatee. He was a pipe smoker, dignified, very quiet and reserved. You had to come to *him*," recalled Ferguson. "But he was easy on the smile and interested in how I had modified his transorbital. Only he warned me about being too enthusiastic."

It's hard to say to what extent Ferguson's bolder operation improved upon the transorbital lobotomy of Walter Freeman. But this is for sure: Ferguson went Freeman one better in demonstrating that lobotomies were a last resort and the end of the line. The average duration of illness of schizophrenics upon whom he operated was 11 years. His aim was to get them into the reality of the world around them.

Ferguson's patients were idle, chronically disturbed or apathetic to the extent of being unconscious. They were patients who daily soiled themselves and regularly stripped off and destroyed their clothing. They were combative and assaultive. Many of them screamed incessantly and were intolerant to sedation, so that it was useless. They were apprehensive of their food being poisoned. They were, many of them, suicidal, sharing in no activities, either trapped in a stupor or "chronic elopers."

For the rehabilitation of this population, Jack's goal was modest: get them better so that they might be discharged home to their relatives; or to get them manageable though remaining institutionalized. To accomplish this Ferguson could learn from the work of others. By mass lobotomies Dr. P. J. Schrader had quieted down the disturbed wards of the Farmington, Missouri, state hospital and had sent a third of its inmates back home.

Yet Ferguson had his own originality. He was, as it were, a psychosurgical desperado. For example: upon certain far-gone patients, the Freeman standard transorbital lobotomy had failed; then Ferguson and his colleagues drilled holes in their skulls and performed the original, Moniz-Freeman operation. The patients stayed crazy. Then Ferguson had at them again with the wide-slashing transorbital lobotomy developed at Logansport—up into their brains through the roof of their eye sockets. And certain of these victims had gone home, sane.

It must be said that Ferguson is not known as a statistician. Though statistics certainly have their place in medicine, they can also be used erroneously. Statistics as instruments can propagate medical as well as other lies. For Ferguson, at any rate, it was plain enough that if other treatments had utterly failed, then there must be some virtue to a given remedy. That is, if it helps a patient desperately, chronically, invincibly sick and un-helped by all previous treatments. This is his simple philosophy, and it is the country doctor in Ferguson and it is also the honesty in him.

By 1954, more than 400 lobotomies had been done at Logansport State Hospital, and the psychosurgical team of John A. Hetherington, E. Rogers Smith, John A. Larson and John T. Ferguson was going like a house afire. Furthermore, Ferguson's recovery from his mental illness seemed solid.

Now his success would get him into another type of trouble.

THE MISSING PIECE

"**E**very Damn Thing is your own fault," Ernest Hemingway once said, "if you're any good."

It would have taken a savvier man than Jack Ferguson to see the trouble coming for him at Logansport State Hospital. The psychosurgical team had no sooner got really rolling on the new, swift and safe transorbitals—calming many violently insane, hopelessly chronic schizophrenics and sending a lot of them back home to their families and some of them back to earning their living—than a voice from above said, "Whoa there!"

That voice was the head man of the hospital: Ferguson and his team were doing too many lobotomies. Ferguson was dumbfounded when he got word that candidates for the operation must be selected more carefully.

But why, he wondered? Was it because the head man, as a custodian, feared they'd pretty soon empty the asylum, endangering his job? No, it was nothing as simple as that. Ferguson was working on a straight salary and was in no way enriched by the increasing number of operations. But this was not the case for the outside specialists who made up the psychosurgical team.

These highly skilled physicians had their own private practices. Then, in addition, they received fees, so much per lobotomy, for their psychosurgical work at Logansport. This was all very legal. But the bottom line was that the operations were making outside consultants more money than the head man himself. That left Ferguson caught in the middle.

DR. ELMER L. HENDERSON had a word for what was at the root of Ferguson's trouble at Logansport: envy. "Professional jealousy is what's wrong with American medicine," said Elmer.

Up to the moment his lobotomy project was essentially censored, Ferguson had been sure—and so had his wife Mary—that he had crossed the Rubicon of his own mental illness. Mary worried that this setback would again send him over the edge. Ferguson was still driving to Indianapolis and back once a month for talks with Dr. Palmer Gallup, but it was Mary who was his frontline doctor. She saw him every day.

Ferguson's success with the transorbitals, helping hundreds of those poor insane derelicts—this had given her husband a tremendous boost. He was helping people again. But suddenly he was caught in the middle of a dishonest power struggle, and to Ferguson's way of thinking, it was his patients who would suffer.

By his accounting, the lobotomies worked. Night after night he pored over the records, the case histories of hundreds of his patients once considered hopeless only to be improved—and in many cases sent home—because of the lobotomy.

During this adventure of jamming ice picks into sick brains, the operation had been tried for 16 different so-called mental diseases—16 diagnostic classifications. It was plain that classifications themselves hadn't helped Ferguson choose suitable candidates for lobotomy. From their manic wildness, their melancholic depression, their animal dirtiness and destructiveness, their babbling verbigerations, their hebephrenic gigglings, their catatonic rigidity, their deadly assaultiveness—Ferguson had tried to sort them all out as candidates.

There had been a lot of psychiatric argument about a lobotomy being good for tension states and agitated depressions and less effective in chronic schizophrenias, and so on. But when the lobotomies helped patients, no matter what the name of their lunacy, it always did the same thing: no matter what the diagnosis, what the lobotomy did, when it worked, was calm them, quiet down their over-activity, make it easier for them to live with themselves and others.

What it did was change the patients' *behavior* for the better. For psychiatric savants, this might be too simple. But for Jack Ferguson, it opened up a new world.

IN 1954, AT LOGANSPORT, lobotomies were Ferguson's primary weapon in his war against mental illness—abnormal behavior. Ferguson knew the procedure wasn't perfect. "In those days," he said, "I thought it was a victory for the lobotomy if the patient could fry an egg without breaking the yolk."

According to Ferguson's own records, lobotomies seemed most helpful to overactive lunatics, irrational and sometimes violent psychotics who could not control their impulses. But the biggest problem with the operation—a problem that always bothered Ferguson—was not what they gave back to a patient but what it took away.

Morale.

"It's the highest quality of a human being," wrote Freeman. "A child doesn't have it. Neither does an old man. Nor does a sick man. Nor does a bored man. Morale is the most elevated of the functions of personality."

Freeman's operation, which had lifted so many insane out of their dreadful demoralization, left patients without the ability of putting group interest ahead of self-interest. They also destroyed what's most glorious about human beings—irreversibly.

The fateful sweep of the ice pick cuts the fibers connecting the front lobes of the brain with the thalamus, caused a particular nucleus of brain cells in the so-called powerhouse of emotions, the thalamus, to degenerate. Permanently. The slash of the ice pick disables things, too, in the frontal lobes of the brain that are supposed to enable you to imagine, to foresee, to think ahead.

Facing these stern facts, Ferguson—himself ripe for the ice pick only two years before in 1954—said a little prayer of thanks. If he could have mixed up the old and new Jack Ferguson in time, so they could both exist simultaneously, the present sane Dr. Ferguson would have certainly slashed into the brain of the formerly demented Dr. Ferguson. That would have killed any hope of the development of the present Dr. Ferguson's creative imagination. That would have ruined, too, the emotional drive that sparked his imagination.

The idea of a lobotomy struck home to him personally. Restoring good behavior to the old, bad Jack Ferguson would have killed the new Jack, a man against insanity. Jack asked himself: *Would he have wanted to live out his life as a placid, contented, lobotomized Ferdinand the Bull? No. Then, what right did he have to inflict such a fate on anybody?*

Only the desperate sadness of incurable insanity that is worse than death, only that justified this gouging into sick brains. Yet the kindly country doctor grew to hate lobotomies. "But I guess God must have had his arm round my shoulder," said Jack, recalling his final days at Logansport.

"AT THIS VERY TIME," EXPLAINED FERGUSON, "we were beginning to hear rumblings of a new drug, Rauwolfia. I read how a Dr. Wilkins of Boston said it was psychotherapy, in pill form."

Rauwolfia wasn't so much a sedative, as barbiturates generally are sedatives. Rauwolfia didn't primarily calm you by turning you into a zombie. Rauwolfia (though ancient in India) was something new in pharmacology. It was a *tranquilizer*.

Rauwolfia pills worked on the thalamus. They cut down the output of kilowatts from the thalamus powerhouse in the brain. The Rauwolfia pills were, in a way, a kind of chemical lobotomy with a tremendous difference: the Rauwolfia pills performed a temporary lobotomy that was not, inevitably, destructive. With no danger of bringing on convulsions or abusive and obscene language or an uninhibited sexual drive or obnoxious mannerisms or a permanent vegetable existence—all occasional consequences of the lobotomy—Rauwolfia pills, acting on the thalamus, gentled the emotions. They did not destroy them beyond recall.

Ferguson obtained 15,000 Rauwolfia pills—sold under the trade name *Serpasil*—from a salesman for Ciba Pharmaceutical products and began experimenting with them. "We found these Serpasils worked better than lobotomies on disturbed patients," recalled Ferguson, "so we pushed for them, only to be met with administrative resistance, even though the pills allowed us to treat patients more like humans."

This seemingly mild remark will have meaning only to those readers acquainted with what goes on in an old-fashioned insane asylum.

At that time, Ferguson's service included—besides his hundreds of post-lobotomy patients—the chronic wards, including two female "disturbed wards" for patients so bad that doctors commonly referred to them as "the bottom of the barrel." These wards were built in the form of a T, with bars of an iron grille closing off the ends of the T from the center.

"I felt those patients should be treated more like humans," said Ferguson, "so I took down those grilles only to have all the attendants petition the head man saying they'd quit unless I was taken off the service and the grilles replaced."

The head man called Jack in and ordered him to apologize to the attendants—or else.

"I knew I was right. I had to treat the patients more humanely," said Ferguson. "To have had to stop now would have killed me. So I ate crow and apologized, but I also succeeded in getting every one of them to go along with leaving down the grilles as a trial."

By doubling their human attention to the wretches on those two terrible wards, pretty soon they had enough patients well enough so that the equivalent of the population of one whole ward could maneuver to the main dining room for dinner. "The first time the gates to the dining room were opened," recalled Ferguson, "it was like walking the last mile. It was the first time in years for many of the patients, and I saw something wonderful. As it came time for the patients to go to the dining room, the attendants who'd wanted me fired had ceremoniously stationed themselves all along the route."

Ferguson still practiced lobotomies, but more sparingly. Combined with the Serpasil, the surgeries proved even more successful. Many times, the Serpasil combined with Ferguson's growing attention to tender loving care was enough to yield positive results. But then Ferguson's supply of Serpasil dried up. Or, rather, the hospital inexplicably stopped providing money for the drug. Ferguson had had enough and began looking for work at a hospital that would allow him the freedom to test the new direction his work was taking. He found the perfect place in Traverse City, Michigan.

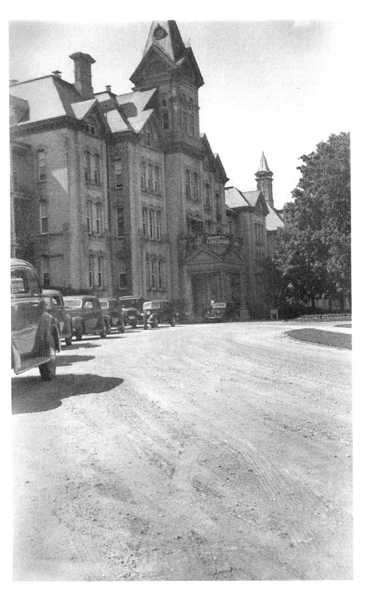

Building 50, 1938.

THE BIRTH OF CHEMICAL THERAPY

W hat Ferguson discovered brought him front-page headlines and solid scientific recognition in just a little more than a year after he arrived at the Traverse City State Hospital. Like a fighter picking himself up off the floor at the count of nine, and then going on to win a battle, Ferguson had fallen to the point of losing everything—even his mind—but now the momentum of his life had shifted. In Traverse City, he was working with a new, cool, clear-headed sanity.

In Ferguson there was a determination to make that change. But, like Fyodor Dostoevsky, he also had a bit of luck. Dostoevsky had his Anna to pull him out of his curse of gambling so he could go on to write his great book *The Brothers Karamazov*. Ferguson had his wife, Mary.

"The first time Mary and I went to Traverse City," he recalled, "we drove around the hospital grounds. Everything was neat and the buildings were well-kept and painted."

They turned in among the many-spired, yellow brick, old, immaculate buildings where more than 3,000 people were crazy and sad. Ferguson saw a crew of patients working on the lawn. He and Mary stopped to watch them. First one and

A MAN AGAINST INSANITY

then another would do something wrong, or fail to do something right. It was curious the way their attendant went to each one, not bawling him out. Just helping him. As if each one was human.

Inside the buildings, there was cleanliness everywhere, far different than what Ferguson left only eight hours before. He saw wards housing extremely disturbed patients, wards that should have been dirty but weren't. Everywhere he looked, patients were neat and clean and there was variety to their dress. Back in Indiana, the hospital dress was the same dress for each patient, as if they were convicts.

Talking to Dr. Sheets, the hospital's superintendent, was like coming into a new world for Jack Ferguson. You could tell Dr. Sheets had a heart for the patients, all of them, the worst of them, as if they were still human but had only lost their way. In him there seemed none of what we so often feel toward mental patients—that they're even worse than animals—a feeling that's understandable because they're so exasperating.

Dr. Sheets apologized that there was no important therapy going on at the hospital, not in the sense of its being able to empty the institution or even reduce its population. He told Ferguson the budget wouldn't allow for buying the new tranquilizing medicines that were just then beginning to stir up psychiatric excitement. But, he continued, Ferguson was welcome to go ahead with his lobotomy program; there were hundreds of chronic, agitated, hopeless at the hospital that Dr. Sheets himself would screen to prepare for it.

"Dr. Sheets was a doctor's doctor," remembered Ferguson, "a soft-spoken gentleman. After talking to him, we were halfway moved to Traverse City."

THERE WAS SOMETHING IN THE ATMOSPHERE of the Traverse City hospital that set it off from other mental hospitals Ferguson had seen, or lived in as a patient. Insanity was all pervading, but the inmates were so neat, so clean. How could they stay so tidy and well dressed?

During his tour, Ferguson kept asking the nurse attendants about it until he realized that they themselves were the answer. It was their own morale. The nurses had no magic medicines. What they had to give these wild, sullen, dangerous sufferers was not science. What they had to give was kindness and understanding. They did not get furious at their charges when they became assaultive; they were not exasperated with the patients when they soiled themselves. Again and again, when some patients kept ripping off their clothes, they did not get angry when they had to dress them again, repeatedly. Their patience was out of this world.

This was at the bottom of the dedication of these nurse attendants: they knew the sufferers were sick. Maybe, thought Ferguson, these nurses are making their own expiations.

On his tour through the hospital, the nurse attendants watched Ferguson's inspection. Through the grapevine, the nurses had heard that here was a psychosurgeon who was supposed to be good at actually cutting insanity out of a lot of formerly hopeless people.

"As good as they were about dealing with the patients," Ferguson remembered, "I felt those nurses were silently asking us, begging me to come to Traverse City and hurry up and get to work."

SO HERE IN THE KINDLY atmosphere of the yellow-brick buildings on the pleasant hillside looking out toward the blue

of Lake Michigan's water, the scene was set for Jack Ferguson
to begin his battle against the Goliath of insanity. But almost
immediately, he found himself muddled in a dilemma. It was
the old lobotomy question. Ferguson was torn, no longer
convinced that the operation was the answer to curing the
mentally ill.

The 500-odd patients upon whom Ferguson had the green
light to operate on were labeled schizophrenic. But Ferguson-
had begun to doubt that his ice pick was going to be the final
answer for schizophrenias. His experiments with Serpasil
had cleared many heads that lobotomies had left addled; they
were a form of chemical lobotomy—albeit temporary—while
his ice pick operation permanently destroyed parts of the
brain that could not be put back. So here was Jack's dilemma:
although he was a lobotomy expert, by his instincts Ferguson
was already a chemical clinician. No sooner had he arrived in
Traverse City than news came from France of another, more
powerful, tranquilizer than Serpasil.

In chemical shorthand, it was called "chlorpromazine," but
was available in America under the trade name "Thorazine"
and put out by the American pharmaceutical house of Smith,
Kline and French. Synthesized by organic chemical wizards
of the house of Rhone-Poulenc in Paris, Thorazine was tested
by Professor J. E. Stachlin, from the psychiatric clinic in
Basel, Switzerland, who reported that its use enabled half of
the inmates to leave the asylum.

Serpasil and Thorazine were under exciting clinical investi-
gation by hundreds of Canadian and American physicians, all
with the hope that one or the other of these amazing drugs—
or better still, both of them used together—might begin to
empty our insane asylums. But for Ferguson, way up alone on
the shore of Grand Traverse Bay, the drugs weren't available;

presumably because the Traverse City State Hospital couldn't afford them.

"WHILE I WAS SCREENING Traverse City State Hospital patients to see if a lobotomy might help them, and while I was waiting for lobotomy equipment to come," recalled Ferguson. "I stumbled upon a small supply of Serpasil and Thorazine in the hospital pharmacy." The bottles of the tablets of the new tranquilizers were lying in the pharmacy getting ready to gather dust, and immediately Ferguson requisitioned and began using them. "Then I found each staff member had a supply of samples," Ferguson went on. "I conned each one of them, and then I began getting refills from Ciba and SKF salesmen. I was in business."

If he asked permission from his fellow staff members to set off with him on his odd chemical enterprise, he never mentioned it. Ferguson was a lone-wolf schemer. Working alone, at any rate, he did not need to argue his method. His chemical enterprise was odd because he refused to try the new tranquilizing pills on any but the hopelessly crazy. He wanted to get them back toward becoming lucid. But why?

To Ferguson's way of thinking—and many other prominent doctors agreed with him—the earlier, more mildly insane are not clear-cut material for treatment experiments. They do not give you a strong enough contrast of before and after. You cannot see that contrast by getting *somewhat* crazy people a little more sane. Instead, you can determine the merit of a treatment better by trying to get chronic severely insane people out of their deep illness and slowly on their way back to sanity.

So in the autumn of 1954, Ferguson began the business of testing the effect of Serpasil and Thorazine on the bad behavior of the worst and longest and most invincibly, horribly behaved among the 1,003 crazy ladies on his service at Traverse City. He hadn't a resident or an intern or any other kind of a doctor to help him. He had 107 nurse attendants who were his hands, his ears, his eyes. They were wonderful, recalled Ferguson, because they had cared for these patients for years, and had been tender to them, and loved them through thick and thin—through times of screaming, depression, elation and suddenly destructiveness, suicidal attempts and even moments of deadly danger.

The 107 women attendants knew the quirks and the moods and the hates and the inner anguish of all of the patients as their abnormal behavior shifted and changed from day to day and hour to hour. All this they recorded on the behavior charts that Ferguson had designed for his lobotomy patients at Logansport. Three times a day, the nurse attendants stood by to see that all patients actually swallowed their medicines, then recorded the doses in so many milligrams. Or three times a day, they put the medicine into the meals of the many patients who could not be induced to take any pill at all. And they saw to it that these meals were eaten.

Meanwhile, Ferguson was watching for the tranquil soothing promise of Serpasil and Thorazine, while his sharp-eyed nurse attendants administered the drugs to more and more hundreds of incurably insane patients. At this stage in his experiment, Ferguson concentrated on Serpasil rather than Thorazine because of its occasional dangerous side effects.

Both of these medicines were subtle effective tranquilizers. They especially calmed down the patients who behaved "over actively"—wildly restless, nasty, and aggressive. They quieted even the worst ones, the ones whose abnormal behavior was measured by the number of strong-armed male nurse attendants who had to be called in to pin them down and calm them when they went berserk. Under the medicines, many of them became meek as lambs, and the disturbed wards at times seemed as safe and quiet as a church. Of course, this was nothing new, since this Serpasil effect had been reported by Dr. A. A. Sainz at Iowa City and Dr. Nathan S. Kline at Rockland County State Hospital in New York, and by Drs. Noce, Williams and Rapaport at Modesto, California. The Thorazine effect had also been reported by many European psychiatrists and by Americans beginning with Dr. H. E. Lehmann of Montreal.

But now as the tranquilizing treatment transformed the atmosphere at Traverse City State Hospital, something ominous, something sad about Serpasil (and Thorazine, too) began to disturb Ferguson and his nurse attendants.

Serpasil was harmless, or seemed to be. When trying to tranquilize the most violently abnormal behaviors, Ferguson found it could be used in tremendous doses without serious reactions … at first. Eventually, however, as he kept it up over longer and longer periods to calm down the tough ones, Serpasil did something more than just quiet them down. It sent many of them into a dreamy lethargy, a curious, deep sleep. Patients on long-term use of the drug could be roused easily to attention from their apparent slumber, but then they went back to sleep right away again if you didn't keep rousing them. When Ferguson kept the patients off the medicines, they woke up, all right—to an acute insanity. Ferguson was distraught.

That wasn't the worst of it. Ferguson kept some of the patients on Serpasil right through their lethargy, hoping it would be temporary, but a certain amount of the tranquil sufferers drifted down into a black depression, a melancholia. Then they began to tremble and their hands jerked uncontrollably in a cogwheel motion, as in Parkinson's disease, and they began to drool and drivel.

There was another disappointment for Ferguson about Serpasil and Thorazine: they seemed only to be effective as tranquilizers of excited, aggressive, overactive, insane patients. They didn't help patients who were melancholic and depressed to begin with. They only doped them down deeper into their blues.

Ferguson and his nurse attendants became discouraged as this sleepy sadness showed up in increasing numbers among the 500 patients, all within a few months of taking the tranquilizers. What kind of medicines against insanity were these, that made blanks of people to keep them from going wild? Would they be any better than bromides or phenobarbital? To make the Traverse City State Hospital a nice quiet place, did it have to be turned into a house of zombies? Ferguson faced it—these weren't medicines you could give patients in the big doses they needed and then walk away from them. They saddened some victims to the point of attempting suicide.

Again, Ferguson saw the problem with relying on drugs alone: they were far from cures for the chronically insane. The blues that followed the wonderful new tranquility, these depressions almost always vanished when you stopped the medicines. Then, for a while, blessed calm and fair sanity might reign. But after the patients had stayed long enough off the tranquilizers, they relapsed into a hollering, shouting dementia. They broke windows and smashed furniture. Or they tried to kill each other or the nurse attendants. Ferguson

began to wonder if maybe he should just concentrate on getting the authorities to hurry up the lobotomy equipment so
he could get busy on the 500 operations.

FERGUSON'S STRUGGLES in northern Michigan had just
begun when Dr. Frank Mohr, clinical director of the pharmaceutical house of Ciba, paid a chance visit to Traverse City
State Hospital. Mohr was there to see Dr. William H. Funderburk, the hospital's research pharmacologist, who graciously
invited Ferguson to meet Dr. Mohr.

Dr. Mohr showed Funderburk and Ferguson a film that
had been shot by a pair of unsung movie geniuses: Dr. Earl
and Mr. Wolf of the Ciba Summit laboratories. It featured a
Macacus rhesus monkey, which is normally a vicious animal
to handle. In the footage, his attendant gingerly touches the
monkey with long, thick, bite-proof gloves. After one shot
of Serpasil, the wild creature is transformed into something
gentle, a tranquil animal that would make a marvelous household pet if you could keep him this way under Serpasil.

The film was meant to show the amazing calming power of
Serpasil. But Ferguson was not impressed. Not that he wasn't
politely appreciative of its remarkable scientific demonstration, but Ferguson already knew well what tranquilizers did
to his ornery, dangerous patients. In the wards of the hospital,
this wonder drug was already beginning to calm (tranquilize)
certain patients down into the Parkinsonian shakes and suicidal depressions. Where was the film that would show him
what to do about that?

Ferguson told of his troubles with Serpasil to Dr. Mohr,
explaining how he tried to counteract the Serpasil blues with
coffee, with pure caffeine, with amphetamines—Benzedrine

and Dexedrine—with Desoxyephedrine and with all the drugs he knew that might safely stimulate a torpid brain. But the action of all of them was either too feeble or too rough to boost patients out of their Serpasil blues and back to a balanced behavior.

Mohr listened and had an idea.

SO IT CAME ABOUT IN THE LATE AUTUMN of 1954 that Dr. John T. Ferguson found himself co-operating with Ciba. He now had all the Serpasil he would need for his overactive, abnormally-behaved patients. And he now was a chemical clinician. Ciba was sending him two chemical compounds, and he, Jack Ferguson, would be the first investigator in the world to try these hoped-for brain boosters on mentally ill patients to help counteract the Serpasil blues.

Ferguson was a clinical researcher now, and he began by failing. Compound BA-14469 had been discovered by Ciba scientists in Basel, Switzerland, to have a notable stimulating effect—like that of Dexedrine—on animals. BA-14469 ought to hold the same promise for humans. Cautiously, Ferguson fed it to a few catatonic schizophrenics. It was sensational. It was weird how it woke them up, these poor devils who passed their days lying on the floor.

"BA-14469 took 'em up off the floor, all right," said Ferguson, "but next thing we knew we were picking 'em up off the ceiling." In a week they were really jumping around. Nine days after Jack withdrew this BA-14469, two patients who had seemed pleasantly stimulated began a sinister twitching dance. This was Jack's baptism of fire as a chemical clinician. "Man, I was worried," recalled Jack. "I could see deaths, disgrace, lawsuits."

Then there was BA-14469's chemical partner, BA-4311, much less active as a booster of the brain activity of animals. It had a lengthy chemical name of Phenyl-(alpha-piperidyl) acetic acid methyl ester—which for convenience was shortened to methyl phenidyl acetate. At this time the drug had no great promise of clinical usefulness; Ciba had given it the trade name of Ritalin. The boosting action of this Ritalin was so gentle that Ciba scientists seemed not to have high hopes for it. Neither had Jack, who again, very cautiously, like the country doctor he was, had started only a few milligrams a day on a few of his very inactive, depressed people. In fact, Jack had almost forgotten he'd started the test of Ritalin, what with his worries about BA-14469.

Ritalin had had a curious laboratory history. It had been synthesized by Dr. Charles Hoffman in Basel some six years before. Ciba scientists R. Meier, F. Gross and J. Tripod reported that this Ritalin pepped up dogs, rats, mice and even rabbits for a while. Then, after having scampered about in their cages, they seemed fatigued. Aside from that, Ritalin was outstandingly harmless.

Ferguson read of only one test of Ritalin on normal human beings. Ciba scientists A. Drassdo and M. Schmidt had made an amusing experiment: they had doped a group of human volunteers with phenobarbital so that they failed on simple arithmetic calculation. But some days later when Ritalin was given along with phenobarbital, it was remarkable how fast and accurately they stayed at their ciphering. That was the only human test of Ritalin recorded in scientific literature, and it reported that of 60 people tested, 70 percent of them were "pleasantly stimulated." It was notable that this Ritalin didn't make the humans super bright. What an experiment, thought Ferguson. You doped them with barbiturate simply to prove that Ritalin could bring their ciphering back to normal.

FERGUSON WAS ON THE VERGE OF A DISCOVERY, although he didn't know it at the time. He had no sooner begun to dose his own patients with Ritalin when a couple of surprising cases began to surface.

One day, the nurse attendant in charge of the Ritalin patients came to Dr. Ferguson to report on a patient known for tying her dresses into knots; after years of this behavior, suddenly she'd stopped doing it. The nurse brought Ferguson news of another women who never rose from a chair without help; now, spontaneously, she got up to go to the bathroom. Finally, there was a third patient who always had to be pulled into the line of patients going to the dining room to eat; now the woman took her place in line, voluntarily.

All the changes in behavior were small, yet significant. Ferguson began watching these first ten catatonic schizophrenics on Ritalin. It was curious: they all were a little bit brighter. It was notable that some of them wanted to shake hands with Dr. Ferguson, when before Ritalin, they'd only looked at him with deadpan faces and dull eyes.

"Look at Mrs. Blank," said a nurse attendant to Dr. Ferguson. "Since she's been on Ritalin, she's really changed. To think that we've been having to give her E.S.T.'s [electro-shocks] right along—to keep living with her."

Ferguson kept raising the doses of Ritalin, on more and more deeply depressed patients, on *patients deep down in the Serpasil blues*, and the action of Ritalin on these sad people was a slow miracle. Now, instead of no response when the doctor talked to them, just the trace of a flicker of a smile answered him, a little lightening up of their eyes, alive instead of dead-fish eyes. Ferguson kept cautiously upping the three-times-daily doses of Ritalin and was rewarded with patients who seemed to be getting better.

Ferguson recalled one female patient known for lying on the floor, never sitting in a chair. Two months on Ritalin and the woman was not only able to sit in a chair, but also able to feed herself. She could go to the bathroom by herself, dress and undress with a little help and even go for walks and to the movies.

On patients depressed by Serpasil, Ferguson continued to add Ritalin, and this combination chased away the Serpasil blues without abolishing the tranquility. Here is a fragment of simple science culled from the hospital's behavior profiles:

Thirty-eight patients have been motionless all the time. Now fourteen are moving around, spontaneously; fourteen sit some but are moving more; ten of the thirty-eight, to make them move, need some prodding.

Ferguson had to admit that the virtues of this no-account, gentle Ritalin had certainly sneaked up on him. Ritalin was a surprise, no doubt of it. To get an effect on these far-gone chronic patients he had to give bigger and bigger doses—but what of it, since it was seemingly harmless. Eventually, the patients began walking and became coordinated. Remember the old experiments with Dr. William F. Lorenz, who first removed lunacy's mask to uncover sanity, lasting for minutes, or a few hours? But here was Jack's patients, now boosted back to activity with this gentle Ritalin. You didn't have to teach a lot of them to go to the bathroom, or to eat properly, or to dress unaided. They resumed these habits by themselves. Without training, many of them. All these years they had retained, though masked, the civilized habits they had learned as children. "It seemed like a mental awakening," recalled Ferguson, "an awakening toward reality."

Ritalin roused Serpasil zombies to activity without disturbing their tranquility. The two drugs acted *together*. For Ferguson, this was important. Insanity is more than merely abnormal behavior, and Serpasil, or Thorazine, tranquilized that. Insanity may be overactive abnormal behavior—and Serpasil or Thorazine tranquilized that. Insanity may be underactive abnormal behavior—and Ritalin boosted that back up toward normal.

In the mentally ill, mixed under- and overactive abnormal behavior is like a ride on a seesaw. So what to do, Ferguson wondered? The answer seemed clear.

When a patient's behavior is wildly aggressive, overactive, start with Serpasil; and when tranquility begins, *then* add Ritalin, to keep the tranquil side of the seesaw from going down too far. And when a patient's behavior is withdrawn and negative, start with Ritalin. And when its boosting action begins, *then* add Serpasil to keep the manic side of the behavior seesaw from going way up.

In this way, Ferguson began bringing these poor, forlorn bundles of wild and negative patients toward a balanced behavior. It all sounded sensible if, like Ferguson, you understood schizophrenics to be mixtures of over- and underactivity. Without his 107 nurse attendants watching every tiny change in behavior of every patient after each dose of Serpasil and Ritalin, then raising or lowering the doses of one or the other to get that behavior seesaw steadier—without the 107 of them, Ferguson couldn't even have begun it.

WHEN FERGUSON FIRST EXPLAINED his subtle "seesaw experiment," it sounded too simple. Yet, I was haunted by his experiment's resemblance to a notable scientific adventure of a great searcher, Charles F. Kettering. "Boss Ket" had started out with a similarly simple experiment, albeit with gasoline powered engines.

In a dingy warehouse in Dayton in 1912, Boss Kettering began tinkering with a little one-cylinder engine, his "guinea-pig engine" he called it. The higher the compression of a gasoline engine, the more power it would deliver, but with the gasoline then available, when you raised the compression, the engine would knock, it would *ping*.

It was a sign of abnormal behavior.

With his one assistant, Tom Midgley, Boss Kettering began substituting this chemical, then that one, for the engine's gasoline. He added this or that chemical to the regular gasoline, trying to abolish that ping. Fuel experts, engineers, and professors of chemistry thought Ket and Midg were crazy. For Kettering, the engine was his one authority. His one scientific question in regard to each chemical he tried was simple: *"Does the engine like it?"* And the engine's answer was its pinging or not pinging.

This simple experiment ended in ethyl gasoline and high-octane fuels. It brought the high-compression airplane engines that helped a few brave men win the Battle of Britain to save us from Hitler. It gave us the engines for the transport planes that have made the world so small.

Not long ago, talking with Boss Kettering, I compared his testing for chemicals to conquer the ping in his little engine with Jack Ferguson trying out medicines to quiet the ping, the abnormal behavior, in sick brains.

"That's right," said the Boss with a chuckle. "Now that this doctor has got it down to over- and underactive abnormal behavior, the important thing is he can *measure* it."

OF THE FIRST 25 CHRONIC, far-advanced, hopelessly insane tested by Ferguson for the effect of Serpasil and Ritalin on their abnormal behavior, 22 were improved to some extent; some markedly; some to such a degree that they could go back to their homes. And stay there. It was harder to boost the underactives than it was to tranquilize the overactives. "Yet," said Jack, "the results are far beyond our expectations. Nothing so dramatic as that which we have witnessed has ever been done for these chronic regressed, negative patients."

So Ferguson kept writing to the big research fellows at Ciba, telling them that their tranquilizing drug had bugs in it. He needled them about this wonderful Serpasil that was being scientifically reported from coast to coast to be bringing mental hospitals a calm and quiet, and that a certain number of people were even sent home as cured.

It finally led to an invitation to New York and a conference at the New York Academy of Sciences. The subject of the meeting: "Reserpine (Serpasil) in the Treatment of Neuropsychiatric, Neurological and Related Clinical Problems." Mary was invited along with Ferguson, who remembered being excited and a bit scared by the reception he thought he might receive.

"All of the day before the conference," said Ferguson, "I got the third degree from Dr. Fritz Yonkman and his staff. I showed them our records. Here was the lowdown—Ritalin eliminates the stuffy nose and the drooling and the shakes and the deep blues resulting from Serpasil. Especially when

you're using Serpasil in big doses long enough to tranquilize the chronic, agitated mentally ill." And Ritalin was safe
in big doses, that was the great angle, and here was what was
remarkable—Ritalin knocked only the bad out of Serpasil
while its tranquilizing virtue remained.

What did the Ciba researchers hope for from Serpasil,
Ferguson asked? Did they want it for a few experimenting
psychiatrists in mental hospitals and medical schools? If so,
then Serpasil's bugs maybe didn't matter. But if Ciba wanted
Serpasil for hundreds of thousands practicing physicians
nationwide, these bugs couldn't help but give the drug a bad
medical name. It might blow up in their faces.

"They sure gave me a real grilling," said Ferguson.

He stood up under it, and toward the end of the afternoon,
Dr. Yonkman asked Ferguson if he would get up at a discussion period at the conference and tell his story. "He meant
with no holds barred," recalled Ferguson. "I had to admire
Dr. Yonkman's courage to make such a tough decision."

In the chorus of praise of Serpasil during the following two
days of the conference, its disagreeable side effects were mentioned by many of the 30 men of medical science participat-
ing. But of the 30, it was Dr. John T. Ferguson, of Traverse
City, Michigan, who really laid the bad and even dangerous
flaws of Serpasil on the line. Dr. Ferguson had personally
encountered Serpasil-induced drowsiness and depression in
a series of 500 patients on the drug for six months. But when
he added Ritalin, these flaws were to a large extent no longer
a problem.

Ferguson was definitely a greenhorn at scientific confer-
ences. When asked where his manuscript was, so it could be
published in the *Annals of the New York Academy of Sciences*
for April, he said he hadn't any manuscript. All he had was

his crude clinic notes and a lot of ideas, he explained with an apologetic smile. He smiled inwardly, too, because they'd only invited him to listen. Then they'd asked him merely to get up for an informal discussion. Now they wanted a full-dress scientific paper.

"At the banquet in the evening, Mr. Harris of Ciba and I put the paper together," said Ferguson. "We did it in the annex to the banquet room. I'm happy to say that I didn't miss the dinner. Although it might have been better if I had: the lobster that night made me sick."

IN THE AUTUMN OF 1955, Ferguson was invited to speak about his treatment of combining Serpasil and Ritalin at the Midwest Research Conference of the American Psychiatric Association. His report, "Improved Behavior Patterns in Hospitalized Mentally Ill," stirred the psychiatric world and again made Ferguson the subject of newspaper headlines.

But what made the assembled psychiatrists sit on the edge of their chairs wasn't the novel combination of a tranquilizing and a booster drug used together. It was the kind of patients that Ferguson was trying to bring back to sanity. It was the utter hopelessness of his cases that made the authorities sit up and take notice. Here was Serpasil, so mild a tranquilizer, so slow acting; here was Ritalin, so gentle a stimulant that it was surely exaggerating to call it a booster, the way Dexedrine was a brain booster.

But here was this Ferguson from the northwoods of Michigan using these mild chemicals, reporting their effect upon the very worst behavior problems in his state hospital (225 of them), without regard to their ages, all of them many years in the hospital, all chronic, all resistant to insulin and electro-shocks, all custodial, all residuals. And now this smiling, roly-poly man was reporting in a low, level voice that in all of the categories of their behavior profiles, the percentage of improvement of these sad residuals "was impressive." Fighting and destruction had disappeared in 80 percent of them; eating habits had become normal in 71 percent; night wandering had stopped in 70 percent; 72 percent could now participate in parties and entertainment, and 74 percent were industrious at occupational therapy.

Ferguson also reported that—since he'd begun the Serpasil-Ritalin project—the hospital's staff beautician was swamped with requests for permanents from ladies who for years had given no care whatsoever for how they looked. Now Ferguson and his nurse attendants had a beauty program going and the newly sane patients were learning to use cosmetics as a part of a program of industrial rehabilitation.

Ferguson smiled as he reported a new enthusiasm for oral hygiene among ladies who had not brushed their teeth for years. Now they went about proudly with their toothbrushes tied round their necks.

What arrested some of them—psychiatrists, psychologists, and journalists alike—about Ferguson's report was the boldness in trying to bring back those who had passed a point of no return. Since his new treatment started, Ferguson reported that no electro-shocks had to be given to any of the patients. And he hadn't had to perform a lobotomy on any of them. Where there was once a long waiting list at the 3,000-bed Traverse City State Hospital, now there were more than 100 vacancies. "The combination of Serpasil and Ritalin," he projected, "has brought new life to our institution and may be instrumental in changing our hospital from a custodial home to a communal treatment center."

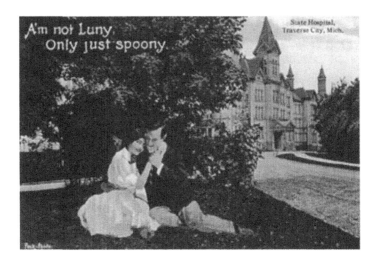

Am not Luny,
Only just spoony.

State Hospital,
Traverse City, Mich.

ONLY THREE YEARS OUT of the disturbed ward of the
Indianapolis V.A. Hospital, Ferguson appeared to be on top.
But among his fellow staff physicians at Traverse City State
Hospital, there were some who weren't having any of Dr. John
T. Ferguson's new treatment.

On one hand, you could hardly blame them. The new-
ly-emptied beds had to be filled. But filling them required
new patients, patients who required complete physical,
medical, psychiatric and lab examinations in the admitting
ward—a laborious process.

Still, it was hard to deny the success of the doctor's treatment. For instance, Ferguson took me to visit a woman
named Gudrum on one of my visits to the Traverse City State
Hospital. She was a nice old lady, well mannered, taking part
in all of the hospital's social activities. She was 71 years old,
and she had been a patient at Traverse City State Hospital for
52 years. Two years before the day I met her, she was hopelessly negativistic and unable to feed herself or take care of

herself in any way. She was speechless and inaccessible. She tore her dresses and underclothes off, continuously. Over the years, she had taken to lying naked on the floor of a seclusion room.

Ferguson showed me Gudrum's hospital records, all detailed and elaborate. She had entered the hospital as a happy, hallucinating psychotic, smiling and playful but out of contact, delusional, asking her doctor to marry her.

At Traverse City State Hospital, they took excellent medical care of Gudrum. She survived severe flu and typhoid fever. She had two successful major operations. But her chart recorded gradual deterioration until, in 1921, she was classified as "destructive, denudative, incontinent, mute, a feeding problem and a troublemaker." No special therapies were then used because for such a dilapidated schizophrenic—there were no therapies. She was sedated as much as possible and locked in a specialing room most of the time.

In 1942, the records showed she had 28 metrazol shock treatments with no lasting results. In 1943, poor Gudrum was tried on "neutral pack treatment," which consists of the patient getting bound up tight like a mummy and then dipping her in cold water. After 420 of these treatments, they were discontinued because they didn't help her at all.

The same year, she was selected for electro-shock treatments. She had a course of each of the several types of E.S.T. for a total of 68 convulsions. At the end of them, Gudrum was still alive but that was all you could say.

Despite all this, the charts said that her aggressiveness and destructiveness continued. She remained nude, and for all purposes, acted like a wild animal. Who can say how she kept on living, or, indeed, why? Yet Gudrum was tenderly cared for and kept alive. Her behavior continued unchanged from 1943 to 1954, Christmas Day, when Dr. John T. Ferguson started Gudrum on half a milligram of Serpasil, three times a day.

Roughly two weeks later, she was quiet and able to remain dressed for the first time in 30 years. Continued treatment sent her into the Serpasil blues, and Gudrum's subsequent fate is really a history in capsule form of Ferguson's discovery of the balancing action of Serpasil and Ritalin on the violent seesaw of overactive and underactive abnormal behavior.

I will not bore you with figures in milligrams of these two chemicals, crushed up in her food and given to her during the year of 1955. Ritalin cured her Serpasil blues, but then she became overactive and aggressive. Ritalin was stopped, and the Serpasil dose was raised and she quieted down—too much down; down to the original Serpasil blues. Then, for the first time, Ferguson tried his real treatment gimmick: after the Serpasil was stopped, and the Ritalin was started, when her blues began to vanish, *but before she could to get wild on Ritalin alone*, Ferguson began giving her a little Serpasil again, to hold Ritalin's booster action within bounds. At last, in April, 1955, Gudrum's behavior seesaw seemed to be balanced—three milligrams of Serpasil plus 15 milligrams of Ritalin, three times a day. "Continues to pick up from this date, 4/16/55," says the chart laconically.

It was as if Gudrum was slowly awakening. In the early summer, she could go for walks outside in the soft, northern breeze off Grand Traverse Bay. She could go to buy little items at the hospital canteen. In July, Gudrum was transferred to a semi-open ward where she actually ate in the main dining room.

"Gudrum needed almost no help except to be reminded to keep her shoes on," said a nurse attendant in charge of her. For this breach of etiquette, Gudrum is to be pardoned. This was the first year she had been off a ward for disturbed patients for over 50 years, and the first time she had worn shoes in thirty. Gudrum's recovery was so sensational that Ferguson took her off the Serpasil-Ritalin. "But we put her back on it on a lower dose to check a mischievous streak that was starting," explained Ferguson.

When I met this little old lady, she was very friendly and sociable, despite the fact she talked very little. Ferguson explained that Gudrum always has to have a hug from the doctor and shows her appreciation with a smile and a new twinkle in her eye. "Gudrum cannot be called mentally well," said Ferguson. "But we are sure she is enjoying life for the first time in many years."

Gudrum was, in fact, so well that she could have gone home—if she had one. The last letter from a relative was dated 1907. Almost 50 years later, Gudrum had no family connections whatever. She had no one, that is, outside of Traverse City State Hospital.

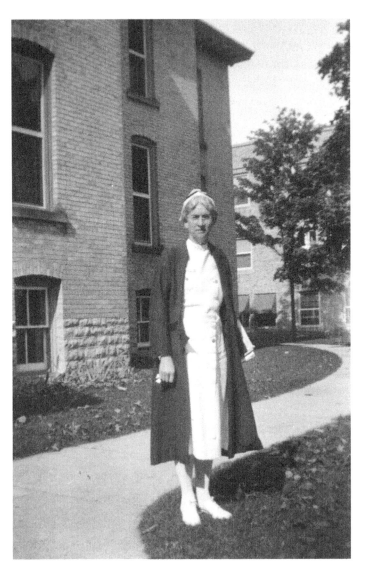

Bertha E. Orcutt, ca 1940.
(Photo courtesy of Fern Rinehart Collins)

A FLASH DISCOVERY—NURSES

Treating patients with medication and love was quickly becoming Ferguson's new method for treating chronic schizophrenics under his charge. And if sending patients home is any measure of success, it appeared to be working. So was anyone else at the Traverse City hospital excited by the possibilities, I asked Ferguson during one of our interviews?

"They don't seem to be," he said. "Their only reaction, so far, is one of them writing to a big Detroit newspaper hinting at my bad habits and incompetence in running my service."

According to Ferguson, his colleagues were prone to gossip and spread details of his less than perfect past. The story about his drug use came to mind. But what was always remarkable about Ferguson was his utter absence of worry—one might even call it denial—that anyone in the world was down on him, against him or somehow gunning for him.

One colleague who did seem genuinely interested in the success Ferguson was having in northern Michigan—and more importantly, how he was doing it—was Bertha E. Orcutt, R.N. The director of nursing at Traverse City State Hospital for the last 30 years, Orcutt's reputation is one of straightforward hardness. She does not smoke, and liquor has not touched her lips. The sweetness of her smile is rare. Orcutt has seen decades of treatments of the insane come and go. This history is recorded in her face, a dedicated one in its austerity and asceticism, carved there by years of disillusion.

"But in one year's time," she told me when talking about Ferguson's impact on the hospital, "there has been an unbelievable change in the nursing of custodial patients on the doctor's service."

What astounded Orcutt—who does not astound easily—is to see something stranger than the effect of the new medicines on patients so long lost. It is the constantly renewed inspiration that has been given to her nurse attendants. "You just can't imagine what a thrill it is," she said, "when hopelessly withdrawn patients suddenly ask a nurse the time or ask to help in the kitchen. Those first timid words are like doors opening, doors opening to the mind through which an understanding nurse attendant may work to draw the patient out to reality."

FERGUSON'S UNDERSTANDING—call it a "flash discovery"—that his nurses were integral to healing the minds of the mentally ill was one of the many things that set him apart. Ferguson believed his nurses should, to some extent, be given the duties, the dignity and the responsibility of doctors because—in a ward of over 1,000 patients—the nurses were the ones who had constant interaction with the patients every night and day. Who better to spy out all the subtle, incessant, shifting ups and downs of behavior?

It's a characteristic of Ferguson that he thinks of himself in no way superior to his 107 nurse attendants. He makes them feel that he is the dispensable one. "If it weren't for these ladies," he insisted, "my work with the new medicines would amount to exactly nil." Medicines, Ferguson believed, were only the start of a mental awakening. But what carried the patients along were the nurse attendants "who poured in the confidence and helped wipe out a patient's fear."

"Fear of what?" I asked.

"Fear of entering into new situations. For years they've been told and helped to get up, to go to the bathroom, to dress and to eat. It's a deep conditioning. They're scared when they have to start to do the simplest of things on their own."

Ferguson believed the best medicine against fear was the love and attention the nurses gave everyone under their charge—the tender loving care that brought back a security long forgotten. To illustrate the point, Ferguson used an example of a female patient who had recently become sane under the new medicines plus tender loving care.

"Except she couldn't get rid of a nasty habit of pushing needles into her legs and, finally, into her belly. The needles had to be removed by surgery. At last, she quit it. She was transferred to an open ward. She was ready for parole and, under different care, she may not have confided in her nurses that she was scared she was going to needle herself again. She felt it coming on and asked to be put back in the semi-closed ward. "It isn't the nurse attendants who first tell me a patient is getting better or not," he continued. "It's the patients, who first tell the nurse attendants, who then bring it to me."

For any other doctor, it would be strange to trust mentally ill patients to know what's best for them. But Ferguson, I remembered, was no ordinary doctor. After all, he knew what it was to be insane.

Ferguson's faith in his 107 attendants is carried to what some physicians may consider a shocking extreme. Take for example, the patients' reports. Ferguson's nurses write the behavior profiles at the start and at the end of the treatment of all patients. They keep daily records of the doses of the medicines and changes in such doses. But here is what's more unorthodox: when a nurse attendant sees a patient getting better, or slipping, she reports to her ward supervisor, who regulates the doses or stops the medicines on her own responsibility. Then she reports to Dr. Ferguson, afterward.

"It's rare to find their judgment wrong," he insisted.

MRS. DONNA PILLARS, R.N., is a 20-year veteran at the Traverse City State Hospital. She is dark-haired and very strong and serene; her dark eyes are a blend of keen and kind. During an interview, she echoed the sentiment of Nurse Orcutt when telling me about the change at the Traverse City State Hospital since the coming of Dr. John T. Ferguson. A few years ago, she dramatically recalled, the atmosphere here was something out of a nightmare.

"A few years ago, in the night, in a flashing banging crashing thunderstorm, the hospital lights failed. As night supervisor, I knew that the attendant on duty in one of the most disturbed wards might have trouble and would be afraid and in danger. So I went to that ward, and there, revealed by flashes of the lightning, all the way down the long pitch-dark hall, she saw women, naked women, standing like living statues, frozen by fear along the walls. Some were prowling about in the dark, nude and ghastly white in the lightning. Others were jumping around screaming.

"Then Dr. Ferguson came and began using the tranquilizers," she continued. "Now, if the lights should fail in a storm tonight, almost every one of those lost patients would be sleeping soundly. And those awake would almost all of them still be in their nightgowns and snug in bed."

The new medicines had opened up an entirely new world to everyone at the hospital—especially for the patients. The patients who had paced the floor and yelled, stopped pacing and yelling. The hair-pulling, head-banging, fighting, cursing and lewd language had vanished.

For the nurses, administering drugs like Serpasil had calmed the atmosphere of the hospital so that now—instead of spending their time cleaning up after patients—the nurses had the time and energy for helping make them well.

"It was Dr. Ferguson who helped us," said Pillars. "He seemed to know that the patients have got to be tranquil before you can make them sane. Dr. Ferguson wanted to know what we knew about our patients, as people. He told us that we had to do more than clean and keep the patients under control. And now that we had more time, we found that we had the power to really help them."

IN HALL ELEVEN at the Traverse City State Hospital, the patients are proud of their two beautiful parakeets. They've named them Fergy and Francie—Fergy after Jack Ferguson and Francie after their beloved supervisor, Mrs. Frances Bare.

Two years ago, there could have been no Fergy and Francie in Hall Eleven—mischievous patients would have freed them, or given them to the cat, or maybe even killed them themselves. In Hall Eleven, in those days, more than half of the patients were kept in specialing rooms. In those pre-Ferguson days, among several disturbed wards, Hall Eleven was *the* disturbed ward, a dreaded place inhabited by beings who were noisy and untidy and fierce and wild—creatures too hot

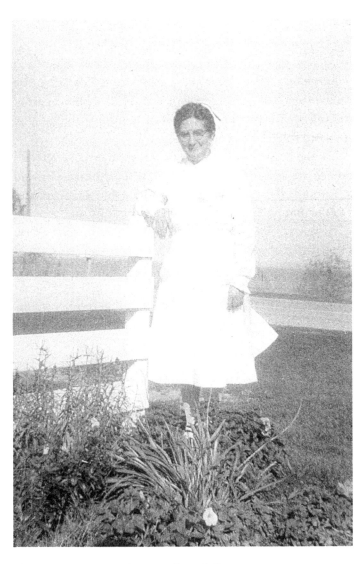

Donna Garn Pillars.
(Photo courtesy of Shirley Pillars Becker)

for other wards in the hospital to handle. Frances Bare has battled against much hopeless insanity, but especially with the demons in the head of a magnificent woman whom we shall call "Dolores"—truly a lady of sorrows.

Dolores was a college graduate with an advanced degree, and had held a position of high responsibility in a Midwest institution until she cracked up completely 10 years ago. It was a break with reality so thorough that the psychiatric professors could have diagnosed her to be suffering from all the psychoses in their textbooks.

As an athlete, Delores could have been a circus aerialist. In Hall Eleven, she once pulled open the top section of every other window and—naked except for a towel draped round her middle—she delighted in swinging, high up, from window to window like a monkey, to the dim-witted delight and awe of those patients fit to act as an audience.

She was an electrician; with cleverly hidden tools, slyly, she kept removing the coverings from light switches—announcing the wiring had been done improperly. Dolores had definite ideas about the therapy given her. When they tried to calm her by electro-shock, she knocked the doctor down and smashed the E.S.T. machine to bits.

Dolores fought with attendants, once ripping the uniform off a nurse, taking the woman's keys, then turning around to present them to another nurse with the remark that the first one didn't have brains enough to work with crazy people.

Dolores had strong feelings about her rights of personal privacy. When, in a search for a very valuable piece of jade she was thought to be concealing, a doctor and attendants attempted an intimate examination of her person. This prompted Dolores to literally throw the doctor across the

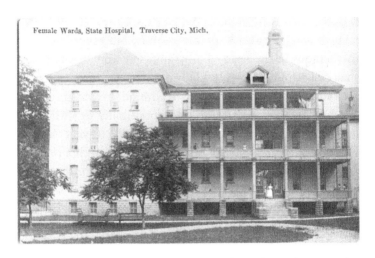

Female Wards, State Hospital, Traverse City, Mich.

room one way and the attendants the other. She was the victor: the examination was never made.

After many episodes, Dolores—who was under the care of Nurse Bare for nine years—was sent back to the halls of the hopeless. And there she remained with Nurse Bare at her side, soothing her and never scolding, while trying to explain away every mad delusion. Then along came Ferguson with Serpasil and Ritalin and his confident smile.

At first, Dolores would have no part of any medicine, so Nurse Bare smuggled the chemicals—they are tasteless—into every meal offered the woman. Over the days, the drugs did their work until Dolores was tranquil.

"It wasn't me at all, it was Mrs. Bare," said Ferguson. "She'd worked almost a decade getting Dolores ready for the medicines to take action."

Ferguson remembered talking with Dolores on visits to Hall Eleven and how—under the slow and steady care of Nurse Bare—her mind began to clear to the point that she began taking her medication, willing. Over time, she was given more and more freedom. Her mind continued to improve until, finally, she was deemed ready for release.

"Now, she's at home, caring for herself, and is every inch the professional woman she was before her crack-up 10 years ago," recounted Ferguson. "I consider Delores one of Nurse Bare's patients, not mine. Just like a family doctor, Nurse Bare was the one in charge of caring for my patients and giving them their medicines. It's the observations of nurses like her that form the basis of my scientific papers, which show how we're changing the habit patterns of the worst, so-called incurable insane."

ON FERGUSON'S SERVICE at Traverse City State Hospital before the new medicines, there were four locked wards for violently disturbed patients. There is only one disturbed ward now, and that is Hall Eleven. There has to be one disturbed ward to receive the incorrigibles, the wild, the dangerous, the utterly derelict from other wards, from other state hospitals, problem cases from the Neuropsychiatric Institute at the University of Michigan and from the Hospital for the Criminal Insane at Ionia—homicidals who need what's called "maximum security."

"You say Hall Eleven doesn't look like the inside of a mental hospital?" asked Frances Bare. "You should have seen it the way it was two years ago to really appreciate the way it is now."

In Hall Eleven, there are pretty curtains and draperies now, and it is a rarity for a patient to try to tear them down. In Hall Eleven, there is a record player and the patients dance— not wildly—to its music; there is a TV set with patients—not distractedly—watching and listening; there is a piano with patients who play it well to an appreciative audience. There

119

are books, no longer to be thrown at other patients, but read. There are magazines and they are no longer used—mischievously—to stop up the plumbing.

"How can you keep it this way?" I asked Nurse Bare. "You still get the toughest ones, the smashers, the wild ones—"

"Yes," she said, "but now we have the new medicines, they don't stay that way very long."

AFTER A YEAR OF WORKING at the Traverse City State Hospital, Jack Ferguson had many reasons to be happy. The hospital had changed. But nowhere was this more evident than during the Christmas season of 1955.

"Have you ever tried to think of a proper way to say, 'Merry Christmas' to a very ill patient?" Supervisor Donna Pillars asked me. "How can you say it so you don't make the patient compare now with the really Merry Christmases of long ago? Can you say it so the patient doesn't begin to cry? If you haven't had to say Merry Christmas to a hopeless mental patient," she continued, "just try to imagine yourself locked up in our hospital for years away from family and friends. One by one they've dropped out of your mail. Cards have become few. At last, you are forgotten, while the rest of the world is feasting. Merry Christmas to you means only a lump of lonesomeness for the lost part of your life.

"And it can be worse than that. Let's say you are paranoid. Your family and friends remember you with a box of gifts and food. Your illness makes you think it wasn't your family that sent them. They may be a trap of some kind, or the food contains poison. Maybe you distortedly think your loved ones are only trying to make you think they care about you when really they've turned you over to kidnappers who are keeping you here."

Christmas was definitely a hard holiday to celebrate at the hospital. But that was before the new medicines and Dr. Ferguson. Now it is different.

In 1955, Ferguson and the 107 nurse attendants—and the patients—began planning for a Merry Christmas weeks in advance. The nurse attendants and the patients beautifully decorated the wards, including Hall Eleven, with decorations handmade by the patients. In the hospital in the past, there were Christmas parties, but only for patients with off-ward privileges. On the locked wards in the past, Christmas parties were impossible because of patients rushing to grab all the food and tear down the decorations.

"This year, visiting the wards," said Donna Pillars, "I did not find one patient in tears because it was Christmas."

Pillars went on to tell how those wild ones, who in the past had made parties impossible, those same wild ones now sat, uncannily proper yet happy at beautifully decorated tables. "They acted like ladies should act," she said.

There was one ward—it was formerly called "semi-disturbed," which meant that order had always been a questionable possibility—and in this ward, just before the refreshments, a deputation of lady patients approached their nurse attendant. Pillars told me of their timid request. "We were just saying everything is so beautiful," said the leader of the deputation of the patients, "it seems as if we should have a prayer before we eat."

I BEG YOU NOT TO MISUNDERSTAND Donna Pillars or Bertha Orcutt or Frances Bare or any of Ferguson's 107 lady "doctors." They are not sentimentalists, or if they are, only a little, deep down in their hearts, with the sentiment bubbling up at Christmas time. They are hard-bitten, because they have to be tough to fight insanity—the toughest, most terrible of all human afflictions. They know there are many patients in their own hospital who could be helped by the new medicines—but who are not getting them. They know there are many patients in Ferguson's own service for whom he has not yet found the right road to recovery. They keep bucking themselves up with the knowledge that they now have new medicines that have started to open a new world to all of them.

For Ferguson, not the long-term but the immediate, momentous fact is that on the 22nd of December 1955, all the gaily decorated wards in his service were thrown open to inspection by the citizens of the Grand Traverse Bay region. What brought a Santa Claus glow and broader than usual smile to Ferguson's red round face was the nurse attendants—and the patients—sending him a Christmas card, written by the assistant director of nurses, Sara Downey.

> *Dear Dr. Ferguson:*
>
> *Just to tell you that we sincerely appreciate all that you have done for us during the past year and especially during this Christmas season. This is the most contented, happiest holiday season many of us have ever experienced. Thank you so much.*
>
> *Speaking for the attendants and the patients and myself,*
>
> *Mrs. Downey.*

In the early months of 1956, Jack Ferguson could look back with some degree of pride. Dr. M. M. Nickels, the acting superintendent of the hospital, and Bertha Orcutt and Sara Downey had all told him it was the nicest Christmas they'd ever had at Traverse City State Hospital. In a single year, they'd been able to send over 150 out of the 1,000 chronic, hopeless, allegedly deteriorated ladies in Ferguson's service back to their homes or to family care. There were several hundred more of them ready for trial visits or parole or discharge to family care or to their homes.

"We're planning a bigger and better 1956," Jack Ferguson wrote to me.

BUT NOW, IN THESE SAME EARLY MONTHS of 1956 when Jack Ferguson looked forward, he saw trouble. It was his soundly based theory that, by the new medicines plus the tender loving care of the staff of his nurse attendants, that he could send a good half of all his incurable patients home.

But not of all his patients had a home to go to. Of the 300 or so fortunate to have relatives or a home, a pitiful 150 of these were not wanted.

He was proud of the 100 empty beds in his service where before there had been a long waiting list. But the census of new patients being committed was rising ominously; and how could he keep those beds empty, and empty more beds, when so many patients, marvelously recovering, had no place to go? Why wasn't the state providing more family care?

And why weren't his medical colleagues trying to confirm his work of chemistry plus love? Why did they seem disinterested? There were services at the Traverse City State Hospital, such as the receiving ward, where the mental illness of a high proportion of the patients was far less chronic, and the proportion of these, having homes to go back to, ran as high as

90 percent. The prospect for the rapid recovery of these less advanced psychotics was much brighter under the new treatment than that of Ferguson's long-lost ladies.

If the new chemistry plus love were started on these less far-gone, and they could be sent home, the census of the insane in the Traverse City State Hospital would go down sensationally. But at a meeting of the hospital's journal club, certain of his colleagues were really rough with Jack. Didn't he see how he was making trouble for them? The hospital was gaining a statewide name for its salvage of the chronic insane and, as a result, the increasing number of this type of tough cases coming in was making them more work in the receiving ward. Although the exact words were never uttered directly, Ferguson was beginning to get a feeling that he had better go slower in getting his patients home.

Or else.

THE SENILE INSANE

It is a nervous experience, this one of making a chronicle of what you believe to be a real discovery, not after the event, when it is generally hoorayed about, but while it is in the works, step-by-step, and with the discoverer himself in danger.

In conversation with Ferguson's wife, Mary, there was always concern that the stress of working might cause a slip in sanity. But there was also danger because of the other doctors around him. It's something you'll find in our very best scientific families—the pooh-poohing a discovery till the duly constituted or the self-appointed authorities give it their stamp of approval.

Ferguson was driven, but the old paranoid part of him was dead, according to Mary. Look at how modest he was about finding a practical treatment for abnormal behavior: he properly gave all the credit for the new medicines to the organic chemists; he gave all the credit for the tender loving care to his nurse attendants.

"All this year I've lost a lot of sleep and knocked on a great deal of wood, wondering when Jack, so serene, so confident, like a somnambulist, was going to fall on his face," Mary recalled. "Yet he kept making all my fuss-budgeting about him seem ridiculous. The old arrogance was gone. He didn't give a hoot about his own colleagues' disinterest in his helping the far-gone chronic schizos."

In this fight against insanity, Ferguson was an outsider. But that was a good thing. Remember Robert Koch when he trapped anthrax murder in his kitchen? What about Frederick Banting, who found insulin in a hot attic despite professorial sneering? George Minot discovered the antidote to pernicious anemia's sure death in his private practice—not at Harvard. Throughout history, all the real originals had once been outsiders.

It's a positive advantage for creators to work alone. Yet, there were other booby traps set for Ferguson in his fight against insanity—namely, overconfidence. Ferguson has had a stunning success helping incurable, chronic, far-advanced schizos. I wondered: will this spoil him? I've seen him a bit high, his round red face pleasantly aglow and his merry brown eyes sparkling at a newspaper headline—praising the Traverse City doctor who says he's helping incurable insanity by chemicals plus love. Will Ferguson begin to believe his own publicity? Will he attempt to tackle senile insanity next?

It is the terminal lunacy of the time, the ghastly opposite of youth—a stage not of life, but of the miserable existence that doctors call "the *senium*." And it's a massive problem, a fact not lost on Ferguson, who knew better than anyone how slowly—if at all—the aged responded to any sort of treatment in the hospital. The sad truth was this: antibiotics had conquered pneumonia, but now these wonder drugs were saving the elderly not for a ripe old age but for a sad existence in madhouses.

IN THE AGE OF MODERN MEDICINE human beings are healthier, live better and longer—just long enough "to create new socio-medical complications," observed Dr. Austin Smith, the brilliant and farseeing editor of the *Journal of the American Medical Association*.

Statistically, these complications add up to the burden of hundreds of thousands of senile insane inside and outside asylums. Each one of these poor old people is a grim beneficiary of modern medical science that has made them live long, but cannot make them long to live.

For these poor old people, medical science is, in one light, a mockery. It saves them from microbic death to end their destinies as drooling dements. Again Dr. Austin Smith peers into the future and warns that as modern medicine lets us live longer and longer, the number of us ending in senile insanity will increase astronomically.

"So what are we going to do to help grandpaw and grandmaw and poor old Aunt Mary?" Ferguson once asked me, rhetorically.

What we are doing, currently, is building more and bigger brick buildings where we can put them away and try to forget them.

In one report, Dr. Walter L. Bruetsch gives figures for the growth of this ghastly army. Admission rate of the senile insane to mental hospitals in 1920 was 5 percent; 11 percent in 1930; up to 21 percent in 1940; and in 1950, about 38 percent of the admissions. The diagnosis is now senile psychosis or psychosis with arteriosclerosis (a supposed cause of senile insanity). These are only statistics, but behind them are people. In countless homes from coast to coast, there are old gentlemen or old ladies. They are clearheaded one moment, dim and foggy the next. In their clear moments, they are afraid. They ask their sons and daughters: "You're not going to put me away?"

"Are your senile dementias that high in Traverse City?" I asked Jack. "Are they going up as Bruetsch says?"

"It's that way and more," he responded, "and it's over 40 percent with us and going up by leaps and jumps.

"Let's look at it this way," Ferguson continued. "These old people are pouring in from their families who can't bear their bad behavior. They're arriving from nursing homes that can't cope with their bad conduct."

It may become, if it isn't already, the nation's number-one medical headache.

FOR YEARS, Ferguson had considered the problem of aged insanity, looking specifically for a common treatable factor. But there were always unanswerable questions: why had he set the dementia of old people off from schizophrenias and other functional psychoses? Why had he fooled himself into thinking their insanity was something special?

When pathologists examined the brains of many of these old crazy people who had died, they found degeneration. Arteriosclerosis. And why not? Of course. Old age. Inevitable. But when these same pathologists probed the brains of other insane elderly people who had died with the same symptoms, they found nothing. No degeneration.

Ferguson chewed on this mystery of senile insanity for years. Of course, it is true that in senile insanity there are somewhat different symptoms. Predominantly, the elderly people are confused; they do not know where they are and they are often mixed up about whether this is today or yesterday or tomorrow or ten years ago. They may remember 50 years ago vividly, forgetting completely what happened at ten o'clock this morning.

Yet there are other insane people whose symptoms are exactly those of any one of the various kinds of schizophrenia, or of all of them put together, but found in younger people.

Nowadays, when Ferguson can't sleep he doesn't reach for barbiturates. "I simply go to work. Work is my hobby and my only hobby is work. So I am up and down all night and can't sleep in the same room with Mary."

Night after night he wakes up after three or four hours of sleep and, alone in the stillness of the night, he scrawls drafts of medical papers in his back-sloping, clear, left-handed writing. Or he draws the hexagons and pentagons of organic, chemical structural formulas of nonexistent compounds undreamed-of, except by Ferguson.

"So at last I get tired and go to sleep."

And now—maybe in one of these insomniac nights—Ferguson finds what may help the elderly crazy people. It is not a new medicine. It is only what he calls a "treatable common factor." It isn't the arteriosclerosis of the brains of these people he must treat. For that, there is, as of now, no treatment. It isn't their symptoms—confusion, not knowing where or when—it isn't these he must attack. Ferguson comes back full circle to the beginning of the lobotomy operations at Logansport and the Serpasil and the Ritalin treatment at Traverse City. What he must treat is what sends citizens, young and old, to all mental hospitals. It is behavior that is so abnormal that those closest and dearest to the sick one can no longer bear it.

Again, abnormal behavior.

And if abnormal behavior is overactivity or underactivity or, more often, a mixture of both, then why not use the same medicines on the elderly people, the same ones he is using to normalize the behavior of the schizos? It would be rugged. It would add hundreds of patients to the many hundreds his attendants were already treating and closely observing. It would mean hundreds of additional behavior profiles and records for him to scan. But okay. He could cut his sleep still more.

FERGUSON'S THEORY let loose a tremendous surge of energy in him. It was not turbulent but like that of a deep, fast-flowing river. It is notable that in men whose energy is terrific under an unruffled surface, there is often an absence of fear.

"The patients we like to get from the receiving ward are the ones whose charts carry notations like this: *prognosis poor, recommend custodial care, typical degenerated old senile.* These are the ones we sink our teeth into. We don't like that word 'incurable.'"

Sally Ann is 70 and a senile psychotic. She has to have constant help for all the fundamental needs of her life. She wanders in the night. Then other patients shove her around and hit her. Ward after ward has come up with some good reason to transfer her. She is too much of a strain for the most loving nurse-attendant care. She has become nobody's Sally Ann.

Serpasil is now prescribed to her and sends her down lower than low. Ritalin is added and Sally Ann begins climbing the walls. But she does wake up a bit though, bouncing badly. Nurse attendants juggle the doses of tranquilizing Serpasil and stimulating Ritalin, and gradually—over months—she bounces less and it is possible for the nurses to reach her. Now she is going on her own to the bathroom and dresses herself. She is caught actually looking in a mirror.

Members of her family come to see her. For the first time in years, she knows who they are. Then comes a great day. Sally Ann gets a hair permanent.

"That was a turning point," recalled Ferguson. "She ate up the compliments."

After eight months, her family asked to take her home. Now she is an authentic member of the household on small doses of Serpasil and Ritalin three times daily and the family giving her the loving care. Her lost mind seems to have come back from nowhere. The nurses and the medicines have put back what seemed gone for good.

IN DECEMBER 1955 at the interim meeting of the American Medical Association, Dr. Jack Ferguson of Traverse City, Michigan, gave a demonstrative talk about what could now be done in improving senile behavior with Serpasil and Ritalin. His was a new approach. The newspapers gave him front-page prominence. Dr. Howard Rusk in the *New York Times* reported enthusiastically what Jack Ferguson was doing to rehabilitate the demented aged.

It seems that our Sally Ann turned out not to be a disappointing "series of one case." Out of 215 poor old ladies, aged from 60 to 84—all of them so abnormally behaved you'd have to call them senile psychotics—Ferguson reported 171 improved, the majority of these markedly. In fact, half of these 215 patients, whose families did not expect to see them back, ever, were ready for parole to their homes.

Despite such results, some of Ferguson's colleagues on the hospital's other services took a dim view of his new treatment. This hostility actually gave him the chance for an elegant demonstration. It furnished him with a controlled experiment—without his planning it.

The 215 elderly insane people Ferguson reported on made up one-third of the patients of this age group at the Traverse City State Hospital. What of the remaining two-thirds in the other wards of the hospital? Bertha Orcutt, director of nursing, reported to Dr. Ferguson that in this two-thirds during the same eleven months there had been no change for the better worth mentioning.

In Ferguson's one-third—after eleven months under treatment by the medicines, always in combination with tender loving care—what happened to their dreaded stage of life, their *senium*? Even the trembling of their hands had vanished in many of them. Many signs of this *senium* were either reversed or were reduced. Of these 171 who were better—Ferguson calls them "my grandmaws"—the doctor was a constant observer. At journal club staff meetings, some of his fellow staff members would jibe him, saying the improvement of the grandmaws was pure happenstance. Ferguson was ready for them.

In test groups of 50 of the grandmaws, he stopped their medicines for a few days. Their behavior slid back into its somber senility. Medicines restarted, and within 48 to 72 hours their behavior was back up to its improved level. Like treating severe diabetics with insulin, Ferguson knew his patients weren't cured. They were only under control. But—and this was important—couldn't their family doctors regulate the medicines and couldn't the families do this under their doctor's supervision?

That remained to be seen.

ASIDE FROM THE MUTTERING DOUBTS of some of his colleagues about his help of the elderly crazy people, another problem was brewing for Ferguson. This came from none other than the very pharmaceutical houses that were furnishing him with research money and free medicines. They wanted to know what was Ferguson doing with this research money?

In Ferguson's service, lunatics young and old were said to be enjoying parakeets, lace curtains, nice rugs, and tea parties. It was reliably reported that Ferguson's aim was to give each lunatic a little bowl of goldfish. Formerly, the nurse attendants had brought their own record players for patients to dance to the music at the little parties. Now, with research money, Ferguson had bought record players, TV sets, and corn-poppers for each of the wards on his service, including ward Hall Eleven. Wasn't this a decidedly irregular use of money meant for scientific research?

Indeed, his modest amount of research money had been given to Dr. Ferguson by the pharmaceutical houses without any strings attached, and the medical directors of all the companies were given full reports on the nature of these expenditures. But what would the committees of eminent scientists, the so-called "study groups" of the Public Health Service, the National Research Council and the great foundations—what would *they* have said about goldfish and apple pies as part of a treatment for insanity?

Donna Pillars, nurse supervisor, had another idea. "Our nurse attendants, working this way with love and beyond the point of duty—that's what's really the most effective combination with the new medicines."

And as for that out-of-line expenditure of research money for the little bowls of goldfish—weren't those goldfish in their own way medicines?

The way Ferguson saw it, if a catatonic patient was given a beautiful little fish and opened her mouth for the first time in fourteen years to say, "Thank you, doctor," that was the best medicine he could give.

JACK FERGUSON SAW a haunting sadness in the encouraging cases such as that of Sally Ann, who could be paroled home as she was behaving normally. Ferguson gazed at her chart. Its heading is a condensation of her life's history:

Sally Ann: #25707
Date of Birth: 5/17/1885
Age: 70
Date of Commitment: 11/19/53
Years in hospital: 2

As Ferguson read he wondered aloud how, on the day of Sally Ann's birth, her father and mother probably rejoiced. Then Sally Ann had children and she herself was happy. Her children grew up, and years later Sally Ann—now an old woman—drifted toward her *senium*, her memory going, her mind fogging, her conduct disgraceful till that terrible day in 1953 when her own children had to put her away. In the hospital, she only went downhill toward a living death.

But along comes Ferguson with his medicines and care, and Sally Ann is resurrected. She is allowed to go home with her family and once more it is a day of rejoicing, though in a somewhat minor key. But there are questions that evoke sadness for Jack: why do many grandmaws, normalized as they now could be, have no family to go to? Why do their children no longer want them? Ferguson ponders and finds no answer, only asking what are we going to do for grandpaw, grandmaw, and poor Aunt Mary?

OF COURSE, ANY ACHIEVEMENT in reversing the senile psychoses of his Sally Anns is a modest one. The medicines and the love of the nurses have not given these poor old people the mentalities of atomic scientists or the brains of the members of the study groups of the great foundations. Or even restored them to the mental vigor of their youth or middle years. The role in life of his grandmaws, now that they can go home, behaving normally and able to live with themselves and their families, that role is humble.

They can be useful, though. They can babysit with the grandchildren and clear the table and help with the dishes. They can darn the socks and maybe even knit new ones. They can set the table and tell the grandchildren stories of old times, even stories of the big hospital where the nurses had been so kind, so wonderful. They can have human dignity, too. They can be proud of their new permanents and keep their dresses neat and clean. Their daughters do not have to worry about them wandering off to get lost in the night. They can go to church and maybe out to coffee with their old friends.

But why does Jack Ferguson work so mightily for these poor old people? Why do they have an especial significance for him? Why, indeed, when he brings them back to normal behavior, only then to die?

Ferguson had an answer: "It's my belief—call it faith if you want to—that now we've found a way to treat and rehabilitate these poor, unfortunate, and forgotten souls. Now we're at a starting point—"

Urge Drug Use to Curb Antics of Aged

Boston, Nov. 29. ⟨P⟩—Use of a new drug combination could prevent many oldsters from going to a mental institution, the American Medical association was told today.

Two Michigan scientists said experiments with the drugs among senile patients in hospitals indicate c o n t r o l can often be achieved at home by family physicians for behavior problems that ordinarily require hospitalization for such people.

Ends Faulty Habits

Researchers John T. Ferguson and William H. Funderburk of Traverse City State hospital made the report in a

scientific exhibit at the annual clinical meeting of the American Medical association.

They said their objective was to eliminate abnormal behavior —such as destructiveness of clothing or furniture, or faulty habits of personal appearance —which predominated in each case, regardless of the mental diagnosis.

The drugs used were reserpine, which is a tranquilizing substance, a n d methyl-phenidylacetate, which acts as a stimulant of the central nervous system.

The idea was to produce an active tranquility in the patients, the physicians said, de-

claring that doses of the respective drugs were designed to take care of both overactivity and underactivity in the patients.

"New Outlook on Life"

Describing studies among 215 female mental patients, the physicians s a i d that in the large majority there was a "marked improvement in the ability to coöperate and a new interest in their outlook on life and themselves."

For example, the staff beauty shop operator was swamped with work following the drug treatments, and appointments for d e n t a l treatments rose sharply.

Chicago_Tribune, November 30, 1955.

"Starting point?" I interrupted him. "They're as good as finished, anyway!"

"Let me put it to you this way," he said. "We've ignored the big labels befogging doctors trying to treat insanity. And haven't we found a few facts on how to use chemicals to put the seriously demented within reach of care, tender loving care?"

IN JANUARY OF 1956, the *Journal of the American Medical Association* published a paper by Drs. John T. Ferguson and William H. Funderburk on the subject of improving senile behavior. Ferguson was pleased and did not mind in the least that the editors of this greatest journal of our doctors made over two hundred grammatical and stylistic changes in his 17-page, double-spaced manuscript.

"Dr. Austin Smith published it, didn't he?" asked Ferguson, rhetorically. "And he didn't question one of our facts or interpretations—that the medical prevention and control of these abnormal behavior patterns in the elderly by general practitioners should be the starting point of attack."

After its release, more than 15,000 reprints of Ferguson paper were distributed to doctors who requested them; physicians who had attended his exhibits at the interim meeting of the American Medical Association at Boston; the Michigan Clinical Institute at Detroit; and the annual meeting, in 1956, of the American Medical Association at Chicago.

But something gnawed at Jack Ferguson: could family doctors treat the elderly in their homes, *before commitment*, when they were only on the verge of having to be put away? Then there would be far less heartache, then there would be far less terrible economic burden of the aged insane. To Ferguson it seemed simple.

THE CHRONIC INSANE

"There's a lot more to mental illness than this abnormal behavior we're trying to treat here."

These words uttered by Jack Ferguson, time and again during our meetings, always bothered me. On one hand, the statement was an obvious fact. Of course, mental illness is complex. But always I found myself going back to the man himself. In the face of the enigma of mental illness, who is Jack Ferguson, really?

He is only one small man, an almost unknown soldier in today's big brilliant biochemical battle for millions with minds sick, scared, and muddled. Ferguson's own goal was small—to bring abnormally behaved people back close enough to normal so as to be able to live with themselves and others. But in today's brilliant (and confused) biochemical battle against insanity, the truth is that more often than not normal behavior is far from enough.

Even if normalcy is attained through treatment, the chemical mystery that underlies insanity is still there. Of this, Ferguson knows nothing. And, worse yet for Ferguson, normal behavior may be only a surface sanity.

While it's true that the sanity of many of Ferguson's discharged or paroled patients seems solid, there are some, seemingly sane, who will tell you they are Joan of Arc come back from the dead or the Angel Gabriel come down to earth. Or again, one of Ferguson's patients may be paroled from the hospital in what seems a state of beatific tranquility. On her own steam, she may have gotten herself a job, waiting on tables. She serves you cheerfully and with dexterity. Then one day she pours a plate of hot soup down your neck and bursts into peals of laughter.

Such delusions and such peculiar conduct cannot make us too confident in the solidity of the sanity of some of these people. But what has always astounded me about Jack Ferguson is that such failures do not upset him. When I brought up these realities, he only looked at me and smiled as if saying that he knows full well that he has only swept away one surface layer of their insanity. But isn't that something? What if it does leave a deeper, more stubborn layer of lunacy exposed? Very well. Now he will try to root out that next stratum of craziness with some hoped-for new chemical—plus his always indispensable tender loving care.

FERGUSON HAS OBSERVED many times that he could calm the overactive wildness of his patients; he could boost their underactive depressions; he could balance the wildly swinging seesaw of their overactive-underactive moods toward steadier, more normal behavior. And yet, despite months of treatment, these hallucinations and delusions—this deeper insanity—tended to disappear slowly, and sometimes not at all.

Help in this next level complexity would eventually come to Ferguson from the celebrated neurologist and psychiatrist, Dr. Howard D. Fabing of Cincinnati. It was Fabing who gave the good doctor his first chance for a chemical attack upon delusions and hallucinations.

Howard Fabing is generous with his discoveries, and modest. He calls himself a general practitioner in the field of nervous and mental disorders. "I have always been ready to try anything on disorders of the nervous system that seems to carry with it the possible hope of success without the probability of harm," he told me in an interview. "Abandoned concoctions and brews by the dozen litter my past."

Like a figure in a Frans Hals painting, Howard Fabing was red-faced and burly with shrewd, humorous, china-blue eyes. He looked like a jolly country doctor (which he is), but beyond that he had both knowledge and an awe of the human brain. Above all, Howard had curiosity.

In 1954, when Fabing was first beginning his work on curbing hallucinations and delusions, he pounced upon the drug Frenquel. Fabing received his first tablets of this clinically untested Frenquel from the research chemists of the W. S. Merrell Company, on the same day a college girl was admitted to Christ Hospital in Cincinnati. She was in a storm of acute schizophrenia.

The patient was loud, destructive, dissociated from reality and was constantly trying to run into the street with next to no clothes on. She was hallucinating, suspicious, overactive, surly, fearful, confused and deadly in her sarcasm. Insulin and electro-shock had not helped her.

Fabing began giving her Frenquel, in careful doses in tablets by mouth. Then more and more Frenquel, which brought this blonde teen out of her living hell. Convalescing, the lovely young lady told Dr. Fabing of her horrible hallucinations that included walking arm in arm with corpses that had worms crawling out of their cheeks and hearing beautiful music and poems mixed with shouts by voices calling her a slut and a whore. Now after Frenquel, these frightful sights and sounds were gone. She became lovely and sane again and was living once more with her family and working. While she had to keep taking moderate doses of this Frenquel, the result was the first time Fabing noted a medicine that was beneficial in curbing hallucinations.

But it wasn't a cure-all. Howard Fabing did further research and found that Frenquel only improved hallucinations in 40 percent of his 115 test patients, which is not bad when you consider the horror of hallucinations. "Chronic schizophrenics did not do as well on Frenquel," reported Fabing. "The acute ones do better."

Since Jack Ferguson did not have any acute schizos in his service, he tried Frenquel on his chronics—some of whom had become almost normally behaved on Serpasil and Ritalin, plus tender loving care.

For example, Ferguson had one female patient whose general behavior was splendid, but was convinced she was the leader of Admiral Byrd's expedition to the South Pole. Ferguson noted how she was also directing negotiations on the location of a proposed jet aircraft base in northern Michigan. In her spare time, she covered reams of paper outlining plans—to be submitted to state and federal authorities—for the reorganization of the Traverse City State Hospital. She was cooking on all burners. Ferguson found that Frenquel tablets not only wiped out her mental over-activity, but also convinced the patient of its absurdity.

Frenquel, in many of his patients, seemed to dispel hallucinations that remained after treatment with Serpasil and Ritalin. Frenquel—even in these chronically insane—was specific against hallucinations and delusions. What happened,
chemically, up there inside the skull among the brain's ten
billion neurons?

This wasn't Ferguson's question, it was Fabing's. For his
part, Ferguson only worked on insanity's surface, on abnormal behavior. Fabing now used Frenquel to ferret out the
bugs in the metabolic machinery of the human brain. What
chemical screws were loose, where was the short circuit, what
was the chemically burned-out bearing in the brain's machinery, what chemical defect led to hallucinating, and delusional
madness?

Howard Fabing is an encyclopedist of the confused and
contradictory literature reporting the chemical reactions that
are supposed to make us tick, as sane or as insane human
beings. Long before Frenquel, Howard Fabing was stirred
by the curious power of a chemical, LSD-25—shorthand for
lysergic acid di-ethyl amide. LSD-25's discovery can only be
explained by God's prankish intervention in the affairs of His
children.

IN 1938, DR. ALBERT HOFFMANN, of the Sandoz laboratories in Basel, Switzerland, was transferring a few drops
of an ergot derivative from one flask to another by means
of a glass pipette. By accident, Dr. Hoffmann sucked a bit of
the fluid into his mouth. Within an hour, Dr. Hoffmann was
crazy; he was muddled, confused, scared and hallucinating.
It took several days for him to get over this so-called schizophrenia. To prove this accident was scientific, he swallowed

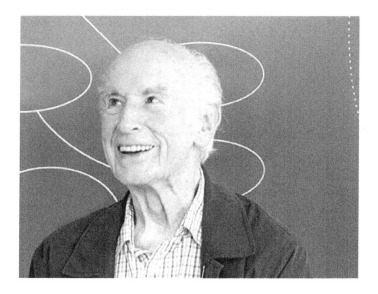

Albert Hoffman, 2006. (Wikipedia)

a few drops of that same brew deliberately and again he went crazy, temporarily but fearsomely.

This birth of the now famous LSD-25 that elicits an experimental insanity, took place soon after, in the early 1940s. It is now established that one-seven-hundred-millionth of a healthy young man's weight, that infinitesimal amount of LSD-25, can drive that person crazy for five to ten hours. Strong stuff. Academically remarkable.

However, nothing was noted about this drug until 1954, when Fabing used Frenquel. LSD-25 is a hallucinogen, a chemical creator of hallucinations. Frenquel, when used in treating schizophrenics, abolishes the hallucinations, which are the spitting images of those brought on by LSD-25. Biochemical philosopher that he was, Fabing asked himself a question. What would this new Frenquel do for healthy

young men—volunteers for the experiment—after Fabing
drove them temporarily crazy with LSD-25? What Frenquel
did, when injected into their veins, was to fade out their hallucinations, their fears, their confused thoughts—as if by
magic.

So Howard Fabing set up a psychiatric milestone. He could
chemically turn experimental insanity on and off like water
from a spigot. And it was remarkable the way intravenous
Frenquel could wipe out the hallucinations of other experimental insanities, such as those brought on by the cactus
chemical, mescaline. But the question was, so what? It was
brilliant and amusing; it would make a wonderful movie,
demonstrating how these hallucinogens could drive men mad
and then how Frenquel could bring them back to sanity. But
it did not answer the really important question: what chemical defect in the brain is the cause of the hallucinations of
schizophrenia? Then a coincidence changed Howard Fabing
from a biochemical philosopher back into a country doctor.

DR. FABING WAS SITTING in his father-in-law's hospital room, forty-eight hours after that old gentleman (also a
doctor) had undergone a prostrate operation. Fabing had just
come downstairs from his lab where he had been observing
one of his young human volunteers, who was experimentally
insane from imbibing the hallucinogen, mescaline. Sitting
with his father-in-law, Fabing saw a strange change in the old
man's behavior. He began talking wildly. He was disoriented,
confused and frightened. Postoperative confusion wasn't
uncommon after prostrate operations, reflected Howard. But
this learned diagnosis did not improve his father-in-law's
condition. He grew worse. He became wild. He tried to climb

out of bed and to pull out his catheter; he was lucky that Howard was there to restrain him.

"Suddenly," recalled Howard, "it flashed over me that he was acting just like my mescaline volunteer, upstairs."

Why not try Frenquel?

"I gave him 50 milligrams of the drug, intravenously," said Howard, "and watched his psychosis melt away during the next half hour."

Frenquel had conquered this very early attack of schizophrenia.

Such was the beginning of an inquiry into the acute insanity known as postoperative psychosis; and Dr. Fabing reports that Frenquel has been almost uniformly successful in relieving some 75 cases of this sudden, mysterious, surgical dementia.

WHEN FERGUSON FIRST began to test Frenquel on his chronically deluded and hallucinating patients, he used it as the only medicine and took them off Serpasil and Ritalin if they had been on it. To all of them, he gave just Frenquel and he and his attendants observed the results.

At first, sanguine as always, Ferguson was delighted. This new Frenquel seemed to have a positive double action. It brought some of the motionless, withdrawn patients who spent all their waking hours muttering to themselves back to more activity and normal behavior. In particular, Frenquel worked wonders with many a wild woman who acted out bizarre delusions, screaming all day, "Get away from me, don't bother me," and banging her battered head against the wall as if in desperation to rid herself of a frightening vision.

Frenquel's virtues sent Ferguson into a seventh heaven, but then came trouble. This new sanity peaked out in two to three weeks, and after that, the hallucinations came back in some 90 percent of these patients. Some of them were even worse off than they were before taking Frenquel.

To any other doctor, the experiment would have been abandoned as a flop. But Ferguson was stubborn. He treated these patients right through their relapses, admonishing his nurse attendants to continue the Frenquel, to get Frenquel into the most wild and withdrawn patients however they could. The result was that many of them turned sane again, but again it didn't last. But Ferguson urged his nurse attendants to keep up with the Frenquel.

And now what happened was better news. The original, first peak of improvement returned this time more quickly, while the setback to insanity, each time, was shorter.

What did these poor wretches have, besides hallucinations and delusions? Ferguson observed that it was the same old story; they had abnormal behavior. Some of them were violently overactive; others were despondently underactive. Ferguson's treatment was simple: keep on with the Frenquel and combine it with other drugs—namely Serpasil and Ritalin—to curb overactive and underactive behavior, respectively.

It was new and unprecedented. Ritalin added to the underactives and Serpasil added to the overactives—both tended to bring back and to maintain the original power of Frenquel over the deeper layers of insanity, the delusions and hallucinations. Roughly 90 percent of the chronic insane who were treated showed these baffling, cyclic ups and downs of sane and crazy under treatment with Frenquel alone. But 60 percent of such upsets were controlled when he added Serpasil and Ritalin.

IN HIS TREATMENT OF SCHIZOPHRENICS, Jack Ferguson is leery of statistics, knowing what he can't know in the general state of our chemical ignorance about insanity.

"The trouble is," he said, "we don't know a thing about the chemistry of Frenquel's effect on human behavior. It's as obscure as the chemistry of the abnormalities that make up mental disease."

So Ferguson asks what's the use of authorities—and himself, too—trying to state, in exact figures, a comparison of patients helped or not helped? What's the good of piling up statistics on a given medicine helping this kind of insanity and not that one when there's no accurate test to tell the two insanities apart?

Ferguson smiled.

"When you try to do that, it's the same as the confusion that might have happened if you had given antibiotics to everybody with a fever—before there was a science of bacteriology to spot what the cause of a given fever actually was."

As always, Ferguson tailored his treatment to fit each individual patient. That way he stumbled on a fact that was to change his technique of starting the treatment of his patients. When the hallucinations and delusions of patients returned, despite Frenquel, Ferguson noticed that he could bring back Frenquel's magic in a few hours when he injected his Serpasil and Ritalin intravenously instead of giving them by mouth.

HOWARD FABING had given Ferguson the Frenquel to fight the hallucinations and delusions, the insanity deeper than mere abnormal behavior. Each day Serpasil and Ritalin and Frenquel, plus tender loving care, saw Jack's combination bring more of the chronic patients back toward what seemed a solid sanity. "Each day is Thanksgiving Day for us here at the hospital," said Jack, lyrically.

I hoped he was right. Where there is great success in the work of any human being there is always the danger of paranoia, no matter how sane that human being is, no matter how modest and how humble. And Ferguson ranks high in sanity, modesty, and humility … but he is human. Ferguson was brought back to reality with a bang.

A certain amount of his patients, marvelously rid of their madness, began to show a new sinister form of unpredictable behavior.

For example, one woman was ready to be discharged from the hospital, she was seemingly cured, when suddenly she let loose a mighty yell and threw a chair through a window. Another patient, so exemplary in her conduct that she was the darling of the ward and beloved by all, suddenly, viciously clobbered her nurse attendant.

By accident Jack Ferguson—or so he believed—found a new remedy for this deepest insanity of all. It was another chemical— "2 - [alpha (2 – dimethyl amino ethoxy) alpha-methyl-benzyl]-pyridine." Chemists called it "doxylamine."

Doxylamine had not been designed at all as a treatment for insanity. It was an antihistaminic, powerful against hay fever and asthma, except it unfortunately made allergic people sleepy at the same time it helped their allergy. In all other respects doxylamine was harmless. You could take it in enormous doses and it didn't harm you except the drowsiness, which might kill you if you drove an automobile under its influence.

Here was Jack's simple reason for trying doxylamine on his psychotics: since it had this drowsy effect, it might tranquilize wild patients who were resistant to big doses of Serpasil. But doxylamine was a contrary chemical. It didn't make wide-awake crazy people drowsy at all. Doxylamine's action on certain chronic psychotics was different.

"This new doxylamine study is a sweetheart," Ferguson wrote to me in one of our correspondences. According to Ferguson, doxylamine wiped out the unpredictable negative behavior of many of the chronic insane, the ones that Serpasil, Ritalin, and Frenquel had brought back to almost complete normality.

With this study, Ferguson now seemed to be reaching the top of the mountain in his fight against chronic insanity. In May 1956, he reported on the doxylamine treatment in a paper read before the Society for Biologic Psychiatry:

The study was comprised of sixty patients whose hallucinations and delusions Serpasil, Ritalin, and tender loving care had been unable to control. Doxylamine faded unpredictability in all. In another group of twenty-eight people, all but three were freed from their dismaying and dangerous outbursts.

But, alas, doxylamine has turned out not to be the perfect chemical sweetheart. While it was often successful in wiping out the unpredictable behavior for a majority of patients, the insanity of certain people developed a tolerance to doxylamine resulting in a relapse into unpredictability despite tripling, even quintupling, the daily dose.

"Has this made you quit using it?" I once asked Ferguson.

"Oh no," he said. "My nurse attendants won't let me stop it. We have over 100 of our patients on doxylamine right now."

"But you were too enthusiastic, too quick?" I asked.

"Yes," he admitted. "Doxylamine is good, but not as good as I first thought."

WHEN A BRIGHT CHEMICAL HOPE blows up in Ferguson's face—as it did with the stimulating medicine that had patients climbing the walls, BA-14469, his practice has always been to admit the mistake, then correct the error, ruthlessly. So it was with the next new drug, deserpidine or Harmonyl.

Harmonyl was the same chemical image as Serpasil, however, it lacked just one chemical group made up of an oxygen, a carbon, and three hydrogen atoms. Ferguson tested out this Harmonyl on wildly overactive ladies, which calmed them down immediately. "But then," noted Ferguson, "though tranquil, they developed an air of levity." They began to giggle and couldn't stop giggling, not even in church.

Ever the optimist, Ferguson tested dozens of new medicines for many pharmaceutical houses. He asked the Upjohn Company to let him try the antihistaminic Rolozote on his chronically insane. He found it to have a special action against the confusion of some of his elderly. Then came news from the Upjohn people that there was danger of agranulocytosis—a serious blood trouble—from Rolozote.

"Upjohn didn't wait for me to find a case of it," said Ferguson. "They withdrew it from the market, immediately. I was just plain lucky not to have a case of Rolozote blood trouble in my patients."

Ferguson purposely published nothing about the famous tranquilizer Thorazine for fear of hurting anyone. Thousands of doctors, worldwide, are currently using Thorazine. It is equal or superior to, some authorities say, the calming power of Serpasil. Ferguson used Thorazine to tranquilize many chronically insane at Traverse City, but he also had a good reason why he never published his results. "Thorazine is okay, *in the hospital*," he recalled. "But it can cause the blood trouble agranulocytosis, which we can spot quick—in the hospital."

The bad effect of Thorazine is rare, but Ferguson would never put out a paper about a drug being good unless he felt it was perfectly safe for a country doctor to use in a small town like Hamlet.

FERGUSON'S FEAR of harming any patient, even the most dilapidated of his chronically insane, had always seemed excessive to me. Did this fear rob him of boldness? Think of the countless, nameless martyrs—not the scientists but the patients, on the receiving end—who have been killed in the name of science on the rugged road to discoveries. They've been killed by Paul Ehrlich's famous syphilis medicine, Salvarsan; they've been killed by the Rockefeller Foundation's now successful yellow fever vaccine; they've been killed by Wagner-Jauregg's malaria cure of paresis; they've been killed by William H. Park's diphtheria preventive; they've probably been destroyed by sulfas and the supposedly safe antibiotics. I'm sure there are thousands of recorded (and many more thousands of unrecorded) victims of bold investigators who take calculated risks with new medicines.

Ferguson has tried to step carefully in his fight against insanity. He was haunted, for example, by what he knew of the brilliant tranquilizer NP-207. "I was just lucky not to have used it during my own bout with insanity," he said.

When NP-207 was first clinically tested in Texas, it was truly terrific. NP-207 tranquilized many a patient on whom Serpasil, Thorazine and Frenquel had failed. The patients themselves extolled NP-207 as a pleasanter medicine to take. It gave them no stuffy noses or intestinal upsets or itches, and it did not depress them. It brought on no washed-out feeling as sometimes happened after Serpasil or Thorazine. It not only calmed them, but made them alert and active. It actually faded their hallucinations and was quietly stimulating. It seemed to be Thorazine, Serpasil, Frenquel and Ritalin all wrapped up in a single pill. It just might be *the* anti-insanity elixir.

Until patients began to go blind from it—until eight out of 32 patients became almost totally blind from NP-207. It took months for them slowly to regain their vision.

FOR ALMOST 20 YEARS, patients who are unquestionably psychotic, have been spectacularly cured, not merely controlled, by chemicals and by vitamins necessary to the health of every cell in their bodies including their brains.

Way back in 1937, Dr. Tom D. Spies and his associates at the nutrition clinic in the Hillman Hospital in Birmingham, Alabama, injected huge doses of the B vitamin nicotinic acid into a dying pellagrous woman who was also stark mad, and cured not only her pellagra, but also her insanity. This brilliantly confirmed a prophecy made by Bill Lorenz way back in 1912 when he wrote that mental manifestations of pellagrins are probably chemical.

Yes, insanity may be essentially chemical. In Atlanta, Georgia, Dr. V. P. Sydenstricker and Dr. H. M. Cleckly gave big doses of this same nicotinic acid to 39 patients "almost certainly not pellagrous" and relieved their insanity.

Even the hopeless, and seemingly permanent confusion you may get from a bad bump on the head may be chemical. Dr. H. Lehmann of Montreal gave large doses of nicotinic acid to a victim of concussion of the brain who was confused and was deteriorating into dementia, and within a month he was back at his job—sane and sound—as an accountant.

Jack Ferguson began to ponder over what Tom Spies and his associates had observed years before. They had not only shown that nicotinic acid is a complete cure and preventive for one type of insanity; they found that an entirely different chemical, thiamine, cures and prevents the mental symptoms of beriberi. "What we are all trying to do is only a first step down the road to finding specific chemical cures and preventives for all other types of mental illness."

As Ferguson began to wonder how many of his 1,000 ladies had come to the Traverse City State Hospital as a consequence of some chemical lack or some chemical warp in the neurons in their brains, Tom Spies sent him case reports of a man whose deep mental derangement had been wiped out and sanity maintained by occasional shots of vitamin B12; and of a very crazy woman, brought back to sanity by a thyroid extract. Dr. Spies reported that he had relieved these and many more patients of their mental troubles before they'd been committed to a mental hospital.

After reading the reports, Jack began adding big supplements of all known vitamins, trade-name Viterra, furnished him by the Roerig Company, to the diets of his elderly ladies who were fairly well behaved on Serpasil, Ritalin and Frenquel. Already he has noted an upsurge in the physical and even the mental well-being of his grandmaws. Jack watches and waits and loads them with vitamins. What's good for their bodies is helping their brains, Ferguson thought.

YES, THERE IS FAR MORE TO MENTAL ILLNESS than this abnormal behavior Jack is trying to treat, and that more is chemical. How subtle that warped chemistry can be was revealed in an eerie experiment by Drs. C. W. Murphy, E. Kurlents, R. A. Cleghorn, and Donald O. Hebb, of Montreal. They did not use dangerous chemicals like LSD-25 or mescaline to drive their human volunteers crazy. They used nothing at all. Dr. Hebb and his associates found that you can imitate spontaneous and chemical insanities by giving people absolutely nothing.

All they did was to have healthy young male volunteers lie on beds in little air-conditioned cubicles. Goggles over their eyes blocked out light. Gloves and cardboard tubes over their hands and arms deprived them of the sensation of touch. In their cubicles, they were deprived as nearly all sensations of sound and smell. They only left their little rooms to have their meals and go to the bathroom. They lay alone with their thoughts in a psychological vacuum. In theory, this super-rest should certainly do them good. Instead, it drove them crazy.

Dr. Jules Masserman, of Northwestern University, has described what happened to Dr. Hebb's volunteers. They became depersonalized. They had hallucinations. Some of them were on the verge of going catatonic—as in real schizophrenia. "Their situation was extremely unpleasant," wrote Dr. Hebb. Only nine of his original subjects for the study were able to stick out their psychologic isolation from one and a half to six days. Then, when released to the troubles and tribulations of the outside world, they quickly regained their sanity.

This experiment by the ingenious Canadian psychologists was, to me, a psychiatric milestone. It goes to show that the human brain brews its own poison when its neurons are no longer stimulated by sensations from the outside world. It

154

shows we carry our own potential insanity within us. I talked this over with Jack Ferguson and to my disappointment he did not seem to be impressed.

"What poisons does the brain brew?" he wondered. "And how many of my grandmaws went crazy from living in such a psychological vacuum?"

AT TRAVERSE CITY STATE HOSPITAL, some of Ferguson's medical colleagues were not ready to accept the treatments he advanced. And worse, there were those among them who were quick to snipe at him for his failures. The same colleagues who cast quiet dispersions or expressed doubt about his successes had never bothered to even talk to Ferguson about his methods, let alone conduct any simple experiments of their own.

So it happened that Ferguson saw an opportunity at a hospital staff meeting. With all the physicians present, a catatonic patient who had been in and out of the hospital three times was brought in. During his treatment he had insulin, electro-shock—the works. He was uncommunicative, dumb, a blank slate. Even Thorazine—the wonderful tranquilizer of the insane—hadn't budged him.

Ferguson spoke up in the meeting.

"This patient doesn't need tranquilizing medicine. At least not now. He's too tranquil right now. Why not try waking him up with Ritalin?"

One of the doctors sneered that he has had no luck with Ritalin used in tablet form.

"Gentlemen," asked Ferguson, "would you mind my showing you, right here, right now, what Ritalin can do for this patient?"

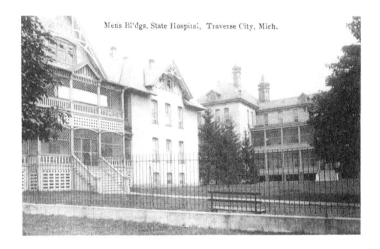

Mens Bl'dgs. State Hospital, Traverse City, Mich.

The medical gentlemen of the hospital staff sneered; of course, they would be delighted to see that.

Turning to Dr. Frank Linn, one of the young resident physicians, Ferguson requested a syringe and an ampoule of Ritalin, ten milligrams, injectable, intravenous.

Within five minutes after Dr. Linn sent the Ritalin slowly into the catatonic man's arm vein, the poor fellow so dazed and mute for many months, was suddenly wide awake and clear-eyed and answering questions intelligently.

Everyone present agreed that the Ritalin was responsible. I kept thinking it was too bad this little scene wasn't televised in color to show the red of the faces of certain physicians at the demonstration.

Ferguson's little "trick" worked because he knew something the doctors didn't, or had forgotten—medicines tend to work more clearly and powerfully and rapidly when they're injected into the veins or the muscles than when they're given by mouth.

From his years working with the drug, Ferguson knew that intravenous Ritalin woke up—in just a few minutes— nine out of ten catatonics even if they were lying on the floor sound asleep and drooling. Conversely, a shot of Serpasil into one arm vein will quiet a manic.

The purpose of Ferguson's demonstration was to prove to the room what he already knew—that these behavior drugs could be used to wake a patient and kick-start treatment, not in weeks or months but in minutes. It was a risky move, but would prove to be something of a big break for Ferguson thanks to a new ally.

FERGUSON'S INSPIRATION

Shortly after his demonstration, Dr. Frank Linn and Dr. Jack Sheets, another young resident, approached Ferguson with some good news. After being resurrected with a shot of Ritalin, the patient once thought mute and incurable had been put on a combination of behavior medicines. He was doing well and seemingly on his way back to reality.

Linn and Sheets invited Dr. Ferguson to come over to the chronic men's ward and stage a demonstration to see if the new chemicals could quickly awaken the chronic, hopeless men in their ward.

Jack Ferguson chuckled at the way these two young doctors had put him on the spot. "Here I'd been boasting I could take any schizophrenic patient who was on the floor and put 'em on the ceiling with intravenous Ritalin," he recalled. "Here I'd been telling 'em I could take any schizophrenic patient who was high as a kite, up on the ceiling, and put 'em on the floor with intravenous Serpasil."

It was exactly the opportunity Ferguson had been waiting for, a chance to demonstrate his methods to a group of Michigan's leading general practitioners with the very worst chronic psychotics they could find.

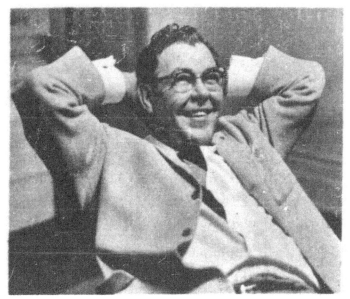

Chicago_Tribune, February 24, 1957.

So over to the chronic men's ward Ferguson went and there he was met by Mr. Chester Krum, supervisor of the male nurse attendants. Mr. Krum knew about the treatment going on for the hospital's chronically insane women in Ferguson's ward and was eager to watch its effects personally. He had with him two male patients. Linn and Sheets had the Serpasil and Ritalin all ready.

Into the first man, who had been catatonic for 21 years, Dr. Linn sent an intravenous shot of Ritalin. But nothing happened. A few minutes later, he administered another, and then another. In between these three shots into the first patient, Linn injected the second catatonic patient with a shot of Ritalin followed by another two.

In a few minutes after the third shot, both catatonics were awaking. The two resurrected men smiled at one another. Then one of them, for fun, tossed the cotton that had been used to wipe off his arm after the injection to the other newly awakened man. The two patients smiled and began tossing the little ball of cotton back and forth. The young medical residents and Mr. Krum were shocked and overjoyed.

"Wait, you fellows," said Dr. Linn, "I'll get you a real ball."

After many years of a living death, here were two hopelessly catatonic men playing catch. Then one of the men suddenly asked to get dressed so he could go into the dining room and eat supper. It seemed impossible. The young doctors were overjoyed, but Ferguson cautioned that this was only the first step toward full recovery.

AROUND THIS SAME TIME, Ferguson was studying *Psychiatric Research Reports 4*, April 1956 (the bulletin of the American Psychiatric Association) and the work of Dr. Paul H. Hoch. The Commissioner of Mental Health for the State of New York, Dr. Hoch was also an active clinical experimenter who believed—like Ferguson—that there was no one drug that could treat all psychiatric disorders. Like Ferguson, Hoch's work backed up what Ferguson had found on his own in the sticks of northern Michigan: overactive, abnormally behaved patients needed Serpasil or Thorazine; underactives needed Ritalin; hallucinating and delusionals might need Frenquel or doxylamine.

Moreover, Dr. Hoch stressed that drugs alone were not the answer to insanity, and that the relation of these new drugs to psychotherapy is one of the biggest problems psychiatry will have to face. Ferguson's psychotherapy—or a most important element in it—was his belief that tender loving care, added to the medicines, determined the degree of the recovery of his patients.

Later, at a meeting of the Michigan Society for Mental Health, Dr. Hoch and Ferguson had a chance to meet. Hoch remarked that he was glad that Ferguson, too, felt drugs alone were not the answer. "It's surprising how you and I agree on things we're doing in New York," quipped Hoch.

IN THE EARLY SUMMER OF 1956, some strange news came in from Vermont. Many clinical investigators had by now confirmed Ritalin's boosting effect on underactive abnormally behaved people. But none had so far published confirmation of Ferguson's discovery of using a combination of Ritalin and Serpasil to steady the seesaw of underactive and overactive abnormal behavior. Suddenly, in the *New England Journal of Medicine* for June 1956 came confirmation.

Dr. George W. Brooks of the Vermont State Hospital reported certain amazing observations on the treatment of chronic schizophrenics. On 386 female psychotics over a period of 16 months, the Vermont doctor had used Thorazine, or Thorazine plus Serpasil, or Serpasil alone—all of these in big doses as tranquilizers.

These medicines had tranquilized many of the patients successfully, but had finally sent most of them deep down into what Dr. Brooks spoke of as an "extra-pyramidal dysfunction." They suffered as if from the dread Parkinson's disease. They behaved in slow motion, their faces were like masks, they were rigid, there was a cogwheel trembling of their hands. Yet, at the same time, there was an improvement in their abnormal behavior. What was this new sanity worth if you had to buy it at the cost of becoming a shaking Parkinsonian? So now to these somewhat saner yet trembling psychotics—still on tranquilizer—Dr. Brooks added the booster drugs, Artane or Ritalin.

Of the 368 schizophrenics treated, 151 were eventually discharged from the hospital and sent home. On this combination of tranquilizing and booster medicines, Dr. Brooks began to be able to talk, as he put it, "directly to the person behind the schizophrenia." Many of the patients lost their hallucinations. And yet, they shared insights such as Brooks had never heard. "They talked about their strange experiences," reported the doctor, "the way normal people recount bad dreams."

After their hallucinations had vanished, the patients explained them vividly. "It's hard to describe what it's like to be insane," one said. "It's something like being in a bad nightmare all the time."

THE NEWS MEANT Ferguson was on the right track. Things were really rolling for him now. His discovery of the combined action of Serpasil and Ritalin—tranquilizer plus booster—had finally been confirmed, and it had been checked absolutely and independently.

Treatment of chronic patients was working brilliantly on both men and women. Ferguson was thrilled. Pretty soon, he thought, they'd let him start treating the less chronic, the earlier insane who live in the receiving ward, and then maybe the hospital's consensus would be reduced! Surely, thought Jack, the authorities at the state's Department of Mental Health in Lansing would look at the numbers and be anxious to help.

In the now two years since he had been in charge of the service of the chronic female insane at this hospital, the number of Ferguson's patients deemed sane enough to visit away from the hospital to their homes, overnight, had doubled. The number of those well enough to be paroled to their homes, *and able to stay at home,* had gone up 600 percent.

There has never been so optimistic a man as Jack Ferguson.

Who wouldn't be thrilled at the loss of terrible mental anguish by so many of Ferguson's patients? What official of the state's mental health department would question the desirability of furthering the program?

Human happiness aside, and taking a strict dollars and sense view, the prospect of Ferguson being able to take his work to the next level looked even better. Every official of the mental health department knows that the custodial care of the state's mentally ill is a big financial burden to the taxpayers. Based on the increasing number of patients sent home, Dr. Ferguson and his nurses on a shoestring budget had already saved the state more than $500,000 in two years.

But a strange thing happened. Officials in Lansing weren't interested. "They never contacted us," he said. "We never heard from them."

SINCE FERGUSON STARTED WORKING in the hospital in 1954, there has been a startling increase in the number of patients paroled from the Traverse City State Hospital; and the number of patients paroled from Ferguson's service is the chief cause of this upsurge.

The numbers look even more incredible when you compare them to larger hospitals in the country—hospitals like Topeka State Hospital, considered the finest in the country. I mentioned the hospital in one of my interviews with Ferguson.

"What's my personnel, in my service, compared to Topeka?" he asked. "Topeka has about 1,400 patients, I have 1,000 in my service. Topeka has 43 physicians, I've got me. Topeka has twelve social workers for its follow-ups to keep track of discharged patients. I've got one-quarter of one social worker. Topeka has six psychologists. I haven't any. Topeka has 362 aides—compared to my 107 nurse attendants. Topeka's budget is better than six dollars per day, per year per patient; mine's less than two."

"But look at Topeka's wonderful record," I said. "The Menninger brothers have certainly educated Kansas people to wanting their relatives back home from the asylum. For every 100 patients coming in yearly, 82 go back home!"

Ferguson's deep pride boiled up to the surface. "For every 100 patients coming in to Traverse City State Hospital, this year, 101 have left the hospital. And mind you, Topeka's figures are based on first admissions, and ours are based on *total* admissions, including all the poor cats and dogs sent up here by other institutions, county farms and private sanitariums. Traverse City State Hospital accepts all mentally ill, including alcoholics and senile."

WONDERING ABOUT the quiet response from officials at the State of Michigan's Department of Mental Health, I asked Ferguson if it could have something to do with the number of paroled patients who ultimately return to the hospital after supposedly being cured. It was a criticism leveled at him before.

"It's fine your number of paroled is up so sharply," I said, "but don't a lot of them have to come back?"

"You bet a lot of them have to come back," he shot back. "But the number staying out, this year, 1956, is three times what it was in 1953, before we started the medicines."

Ferguson explained that 61 percent of those paroled—all of them had been chronically insane—are now holding their recovery solidly. But then he said something that made me sit up.

"We know why nine out of ten of those who relapse, relapse. They blow up because there's no medical supervision to see they keep on with their medicines at home or regulate the doses. They relapse because there is mismanagement of many patients put out to family-care homes. The state doesn't pay the family-care people enough per day to make it worth their while to be attentive or considerate to their newly sane guests. And there is often a failure, or a lapse of tender loving care on the part of the relatives to whom the newly sane folks have returned.

"Here you really get to know the stigma of having been mentally ill," he continued. "People don't seem to be able to believe a patient has recovered."

When patients relapsed and came back to the hospital, Ferguson insisted that it was easier to bring them back to reality the second time. "Now we have the intravenous medicines," he said. "In two days, we can have them out on grounds parole. In a week, we can have them back to family care or back home."

When you look at it from a certain point of view, having to go back to the asylum—if you are one of Dr. Ferguson's patients—may not be as bad as you think. Ask Dr. Raymond C. Pogge, research director of the William S. Merrell Company. This is the company that first put the medicine, Frenquel, into the hands of Jack Ferguson, and Dr. Pogge had been closely inspecting Ferguson's work at Traverse City ever since. In part, Pogge wrote in a letter to me:

> *I think most of us who are interested in the newer methods of treating mental illness are more or less familiar with Dr. Ferguson's outstanding work, but one thing which [sic] I had not previously realized is not really related to drug therapy.*
>
> *I refer to the inspiration which [sic] trickles down from Dr. Ferguson directly to his patients and through his entire nursing staff. Combine this inspiration with the physical properties of the hospital—new model pianos, parakeets, light cheerful chair covers, attractive draperies. All this has made this institution certainly the jolliest mental hospital I have ever seen.*

ONE OFFICIAL FROM THE STATE DEPARTMENT of Mental Health did eventually come up from Lansing to get figures on the notable increase in the discharge of the Traverse City patients. This was followed by a press release from the mental health department at Lansing stating that this was going on at "a Michigan Hospital."

No mention of Traverse City. Likewise, no official from the state health department has ever come to examine Ferguson's work. The State Mental Health Commission convenes three days each summer in the soft breezes of the salubrious air of the region of Traverse City, yet no member has ever made a tour of Ferguson's service. None has asked him a question.

Through channels, Ferguson has pleaded for clerical help to compile his growing mass of statistics on parole and recovery. He has begged for modest money for social workers to trace the fate of paroled patients in their homes or on family care. To this request, there has not even been an answer. But to this bureaucratic indifference, Ferguson only smiled.

"The Lansing people are really recognizing our good work of sending so many folks home," quipped Ferguson. "They've taken the whole Flint area away from the Pontiac State Hospital and are sending all Flint patients to us."

To Ferguson's charitable way of thinking, the Lansing people may have more scientific savvy than they are letting on. "They may have a mighty sound reason for giving the big research appropriations to the University of Michigan and the Lafayette Clinic at Detroit—instead of to us up here in the sticks."

Such cool-headed gentleness puzzled me. Considering the way he and others in Traverse City were saving the State of Michigan hundreds of thousands of dollars—not to mention the way they were bringing many Michigan people up out of years of mental anguish—what sound reason could the Lansing officials possibly have for not giving the Traverse City State Hospital a bit more money for follow-up of paroled patients and for additional family care for the hundreds now ready and able to leave the hospital?

Ferguson had an ironical answer. "Maybe they're trying a big experiment—to find out what the University and the Lafayette Clinic can do with the research money for the state's insane, compared to what we are doing up here without money."

"But seriously, look at it from the point of view of the Lansing officials," he continued. "If they gave money to us, they'd have all the other state hospitals down their necks."

OFTEN DURING THE COURSE of writing and interviewing Jack Ferguson, I wondered what power on earth could stop him. Ferguson was a man without jealously. He hated no human being, only insanity. He fights it with facts. Every defeat means only a new research project. He fails forward, always to a new duty. That duty now is keeping the maximum possible number of his patients home or under family care, to get them back to work, and to the nearest possible complete recovery—once they're well enough to leave the hospital.

With no expert statistical assistance at all, with little clerical help, alone on his own every day and far into every night, Ferguson slogs through masses of records. What does he look for? He is searching out those patients who have had to return to the hospital after their first recovery. His eyes are blurred, his hands are cramped.

"Seems I'll never get this damn job done," he confided to me in a phone call. "Why don't they give me a little help? I've about run out of gas."

But two days later he calls back, and his voice is a little high with excitement, different from his customary low key. He's discovered something after tagging all his relapsers by name, number and the history of the events that led up to their return to the asylum. "Now we're rolling," he says. "Since they've recovered once under the new medicines and our T.L.C.—we believe they can recover again. We believe they're potentially curable."

"It going to be an awful job to cure them all over," I reply.

But Ferguson laughs out loud. "Not with what we've got now. Now we can snap most of 'em out of their bad behavior quickly, by the medicines into their veins. Then in a couple of days switching to treatment by mouth, balancing the seesaw, steadying it by tender loving care."

"But who'll keep them steady when they're out?" I ask.

FOR MANY MONTHS, Ferguson watched patients coming back to the hospital because of faulty management of their medicines. For a long time, he'd been getting a stream of letters from relatives of patients who had left the hospital; the letters reporting the patient's condition and asking: "Should we continue the medicines?"

Like any good doctor, Ferguson doesn't like to answer that question without seeing the patient. But he's quietly furious at a part of his program being wasted because of lack of medical follow-up. Now more than ever, Ferguson feels that a collaboration between the state hospital and the family doctors is an essential part of treatment that is lacking. "When that gets rolling we'll really cut down our relapsers," he said. "Nine out of ten of those who *do* relapse go sour at home due to lack of proper medical follow-up."

Ferguson knew any competent doctor will see the sense of such a follow-up. It isn't enough to give the patient and family a bottle of the medicines and walk away, as is now often done for fighting infections with antibiotics. The behavior drugs aren't that kind of medicine. They're not *cures* for mental illness, any more than insulin is a cure for diabetes.

"Think of your controlled diabetic," Jack reasoned. "If he overeats, the doctor may have to give him more insulin. If he goes low on food, the doctor may have to cut the insulin down. It's your seesaw again, just like in mental illness.

"No good doctor starts patients on insulin shots and neglects the all-important diet," Jack continued. "It's just the same with abnormal behavior. No good doctor will just chuck the new medicines into the patient—without seeing to it that the patient has a diet of tender loving care at home."

During our interviews, Ferguson insisted that many family doctors grasped his ideas when he compared the aftercare of the paroled mental patient to the care of the controlled diabetic. "When a mental patient becomes upset, or depressed, temporarily," he explained, "the addition of a little more tranquilizing or boosting medicine will help the patients to weather these storms."

UNLIKE HIS CONTEMPORARIES, Ferguson believed in the family doctors' ability to keep the mentally insane from relapsing—provided that the recovered patients and their families were taught the importance of regularly administering medication. "The great thing about our family doctors is that they're interested in their patients as people. They're willing to work with their patients and families to help the new medicines. That way they'll keep the seesaw of behavior steady."

For Ferguson, there is a bright prospect of hope growing out of the insight that comes from his experience with his own former insanity. It is actually easier for physicians to treat recovered patients than it is to keep people threatened by heart failure under control with digitalis, or to keep diabetics on an even keel with insulin. Why? Because, in case of congestive heart failure or diabetes, deterioration may go too far before the patients feel sick. In mental illness, the slightest symptoms of a return of trouble are felt—at once—in the head.

As if to anticipate my question, Ferguson smiled and said: "You're wondering why Michigan's doctors aren't routinely helping these recovered patients, now? At this stage of the game, it isn't the doc's fault he isn't already at it. It's all so new. But the pattern's here now. It's no different from what they're doing in their home care of patients discharged from Veterans Administration hospitals."

FERGUSON'S NOTION that patients—under the care of family doctors—could be responsible for their own treatment was fascinating. So I sought out one who was making it work.

"I tried to go through the shock treatments without kicking up too much," Elaine Menzell wrote in a letter to me. "After I was getting the new medicines a while, those last two shock treatments seemed very terrible."

Elaine Menzell had been out of Traverse City State Hospital for over a year and a half now. She had a job and was living a normal life.

Soon after Serpasil, then Ritalin, then Serpasil and Ritalin had replaced the shock treatments, Menzell had come out of her wild, frightened, nightmare world back to reality. Soon she was paroled to the care of her sister, Mrs. Dorothea Schaffer, one of Ferguson's nurse attendants. "I was taking a whole pill at home, then half, then a quarter, then back to a half because we were having a few arguments right then," she wrote. "I felt safer on a half."

"Elaine's explaining how we had to raise the doses a bit around Christmas 1955," said Dorothea Schaffer. "The tension of the holidays and the decisions on what to buy and how much to spend on various relatives made both of us a little nervous."

Schaffer explained that, soon after getting back home from the hospital, Menzell began carrying a little pill box containing the medicines with her all the time. "Whenever Elaine feels the need," said Schaffer, "she comes and tells me she's increasing the Serpasil, and also when she's decreasing it."

Elaine Menzell has become her own front-line psychiatrist. In her memo to me, written with wit and in a clear hand, she showed her insight. "When I need a pill I've forgotten to take," she wrote, "I begin to feel talkative and energetic and silly, and as soon as I feel it I take that forgotten pill right now."

FERGUSON HAS A VISION, but he is not visionary. He is, instead, practical. The family doctor has the new behavior medicines. They are safe. Their cost is low. By teaming up with family doctors when they release a patient out of the asylum, Ferguson believes he can get competent doctors to understand the uses and limitations of the new medicines and the power of tender loving care. And as general practitioners see patients that were considered absolutely incurable—as they see these hopeless now taking their places in the community again—they'll start using the medicines to prevent others from having to be committed.

"The final way to empty our asylums is to keep the mentally ill from entering, or re-entering, them," says Ferguson.

"Couldn't we all try to keep ourselves behaving more normally without going to our doctor at all—just buying these wonderful new happiness pills over the drugstore counter?" I once asked Ferguson. It is exactly this that I myself had tried, two years ago.

"What happened to you, when you tried that without a doctor's advice?"

"It sent me into two bad depressions," I said.

"Exactly," he said. "Then why do you ask me such a silly question? It's the duty of the physicians to warn patients against treating themselves with any and all happiness pills.

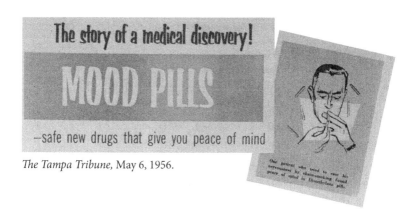

The story of a medical discovery!

MOOD PILLS

—safe new drugs that give you peace of mind

The Tampa Tribune, May 6, 1956.

Who but a good doctor can judge whether these medicines are effective or not effective—against over- and under-active behavior? And against hallucinations and paranoia and melancholia? Would you want weird celebrities from Hollywood—the ones that are plugging these happiness pills—would you want them to prescribe for you in a mental or emotional tailspin?"

Ferguson gave me his view of the danger of trying to self-medicate myself toward happiness. "Let's put it this way. When you buy happiness pills, or any others you can get across the counter, you're in danger of depressing yourself into a melancholia without a doctor watching."

Ferguson wouldn't *want* a miracle pill or a magic injection that would reverse insanity, instantly. In the future, such a pill might come, but who knows? For Ferguson, the mightiest pill in the world would still need love to make it stick.

So I ask him, awed as I am by all he has been through, to tell me just what is a psychiatrist.

"To me a psychiatrist is not a man who simply knows big words or directs the lives of others," he said. "He is a man who admits his own limitations. He is a man who can temper his judgment of a bad act with a form of charity. This gives mixed-up people an understanding that will cast out fear. I'd like to get to be that kind of man."

It's interesting to note that Ferguson is as thrilled by the new medicines as he is afraid of them. "The medicines tend to make us forget that all these patients are human. The way they awake people out of their darkness, they might make you think patients are only chemical."

Ferguson then defined for me the type of psychiatrist he does not want to be like—a doctor who spends hours formulating a diagnosis that is carefully branded on a patient like handlebars to hang on to; a doctor whose treatment is a jolt of electricity, a good stiff slug of insulin, or a dose of Thorazine or Serpasil with all the rest of the patient ignored. Ferguson does not want to be a doctor who does not soil his hands.

"I get mighty tired sometimes," admits Ferguson. "Now that God has given me what you call the moxie, it'd be easy for me to pull out and get me a big-time, big-money practice."

But, Ferguson continues, he is completely without ambition to be the boss, a big-time administrator of a mental hospital, even though he's still tempted by a dream of abolishing insane asylums and changing them into community treatment centers for abnormal behavior.

"I know it could be done. I know it by the faith the patients and nurses have in me. I sometimes think I could do it. But then I pin my own ears back by a little prayer. I say it many times every day."

Jack got out his wallet and handed me a little card to read.

God grant me the serenity to accept things I cannot change, the courage to change things I can, and the wisdom to know the difference.

"Who wrote that?" I asked.

"It's from the AA's prayer," he answered.

"But you've never been an alcoholic," I protested.

"That's right," he said, "I've been worse."

This is Ferguson's wisdom: to know that he is a country doctor who can help crazy people and to know that he is not the executive type or a big wheel who can administer institutions.

The AA card—Ferguson has carried it many years—is his medicine against paranoia. It was given to him by his mother.

WHAT WILL BECOME OF JACK FERGUSON? It is possible that his shrewd tricks against insanity will be appropriated in a disguised form by ambitious psychiatrists. It may even happen that his humble discoveries will be buried, his name snowed under by the psychopharmacologic science pouring out of the university medical schools.

Yet it is my faith that someone will someday rediscover Ferguson's plain science. After all, the honest Dutch biologist Hugo de Vries unearthed the buried genetic discoveries of forgotten Gregor Mendel and then published them as Mendel's, not as his own, although De Vries had rediscovered them at a time he had not heard of Mendel.

But what will become of Jack Ferguson in the near future?

What if Ferguson's new tricks pile up a bigger and bigger log jam of people in the Traverse City State Hospital? Does their existence even now threaten to become a scandal?

SO WE LEAVE DR. JOHN T. FERGUSON the family doctor at his lab bench, namely, the wards and the cottages and the halls of the Traverse City State Hospital. We leave him looking out for his big family, the chronic crazy ladies on their way back to sanity. And his family is growing, for now they're letting him assist in treating the crazy men, too. You remember those two hopeless catatonics playing catch and talking sanely 15 minutes after their shots of Ritalin? We leave Ferguson, growing. Growing to be a shrewder and shrewder experimenter, looking for safer and more subtle medicines.

We might well take leave of Jack Fergusonas he sits on the floor in Hall Eleven by the side of a wretched woman dead to the world and drooling. His arm is around her and he is whispering to her earnestly as if she can actually register what he is saying to her.

"I've had to fight my way out of a ward like this. I had to go back four times before I came out okay. And I came out okay. I had to go back because I wouldn't listen to the doctors. Please open your mouth and let the nurse give you this new medicine. I'm still taking my own medicine. You know what it is, Jean?" Jack calls all the patients by their first names, remembering them. "You know what's *my* medicine, Jean? It's helping you to come back the way I came back."

Ferguson works with every one of his patients; no matter how manic, how negative, how withdrawn. He operates as if every patient knows and remembers what he's telling them. And then, as the medicines bring them back to reality, the patients show him that they *do* remember. They say: "Doctor, you were locked up in a place like this?"

"Yes, five times in a place like this, and worse," he answers.

Perhaps that makes his ladies on their way back to reality understand why he puts his arm around them.

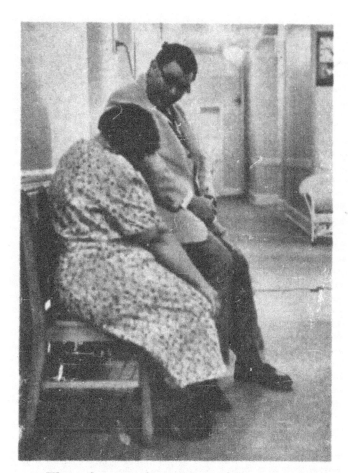

The doctor listens to her story.

Chicago Tribune, November 30, 1955. Photo by Andrew Ravlin.

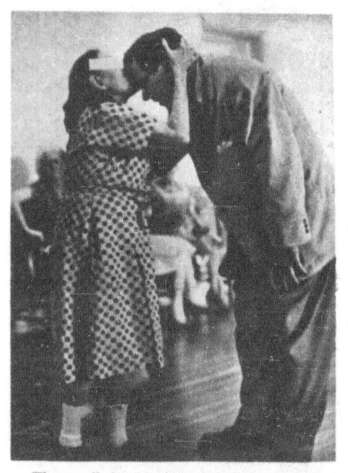

They all love this outgoing man.

Chicago Tribune, November 30, 1955. Photo by Andrew Ravlin.

"One pat on the back is giving them six pills," he says. "I see them as sufferers. As sick human beings, not as animals or test tubes."

In the wards the patients crowd around Ferguson, and he has a word for every one of them. "Now Helen, you just wait," he says. "I'll talk to you when I get through with Jane."

After he has listened to their troubles and told them, as he does again and again, the story of his own stormy past, they join a procession, following after their jolly, kidding, ruddy-faced doctor. And he has a pocketful of shiny new dimes, a dime and good word for every one of them.

"You wonder why I was down on the floor with that drooling dead-to-the-world woman," he asks.

"I was trying to catch a first word she might suddenly say while I was telling her about my own crazy past. Tomorrow, next week, the medicines will really have her talking to me. They all have a language that's understandable. That's the big job and the secret of trying to help these mentally ill people. It isn't so hard to understand the craziest talk. It just takes listening.

"Many people are called unnaturally strange or even demented because they are not understood. History is loaded with them, from Jesus to Billy Mitchell—who was court-martialed for insubordination in WWI."

Ferguson's thoughts flash back to his own days in the locked ward of the veterans' hospital. Someone in those dark days learned the language and then spoke and helped him.

"So I look at my patients," he says. "I look at them and I think that if, here standing before me, was a very important person who could do me some good, it would be very easy for me to spend the time learning her language. But this patient, this poor woman cannot help me. What would I want if our positions were reversed?"

So Jack Ferguson takes time to learn the language of all of them coming back to reality and it is incredible the time it takes him to make his ward rounds. Let us take off our hats to the chemists who invented the brilliant behavior medicines. And will the men of the pharmaceutical and chemical houses who have made these medicines available, will they please take a bow. But the mystery of Jack Ferguson is that Jack himself is the medicine.

POST SCRIPT

We sent the manuscript of this story to Dr. William F. Lorenz, the researcher who first brought about, chemically, a lucid interval in the chronic, hopeless insane. When he wired that he'd read it and liked it, my wife, Rhea, and I drove 700 miles through a mild fall season of bright yellow poplars and the old gold of tamaracks to have a talk with Lorenz, to thank him for having inspired us and to receive his blessing.

Those two hours will be unforgettable. Old Bill, his eyes wrinkly at the corners and his lean face crosshatched with deep wrinkles, looked more than ever like a tank general—like a killer, not of men but of man's worst enemy, insanity. Bill pointed out that we have written of a medical adventure that is only in its beginning, and that ten years from now, new medicines will make today's triumphs obsolete.

"But," said Bill, "please tell Dr. Ferguson of my admiration for his insight and knowledge—and for his courage to have carried his work through to its present hopeful state."

And as we told each other goodbye, Bill gave us this last word. "Tell people not to worry about there being only one Ferguson," he said. "Look at how Jack has made doctors out of his 107 nurse attendants. By teaching, we can make thousands of men fight against insanity, among them our family doctors."

That was Bill's last word to me as he stood by his log cabin in the woods by his lake in northern Wisconsin.

Dr. Ferguson, TCSH Staff Member, Dies

Dr. John T. Ferguson, 59, who achieved national prominence at Traverse City State Hospital for his pioneer efforts in the use of drugs to treat mental illness, died suddenly Friday evening.

He was stricken while helping direct traffic at 11th and Division during a minor fire at

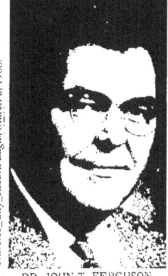

DR. JOHN T. FERGUSON

the state hospital. He was dead on arrival at Munson Medical Center.

Dr. Ferguson was born May 3, 1908 in Monon, Indiana. He attended schools in Monon and graduated in 1948 from the Indiana University Medical School. He was married to the former Mary Tosti April 23, 1944 at Bloomington, Ind. He had been living in Traverse City since 1954. His home was at 730 W. 11th street.

He was a member of the St. Aloysius Church of Fife Lake. He was affiliated with the Phi Chi medical fraternity and was a member of the Grand Traverse - Leelanau - Benzie County Medical Society, the Michigan State Medical Society, the American Medical Association, the American Psychiatric Association and was a Fellow at the American Geriatric Society.

Surviving, in addition to his wife, are one sister, Marjorie Thompson of Denver, Colorado; and six nieces and nephews.

Funeral services will be Tuesday at 11 a.m. at the Carmelite Monastery Chapel on Silver Lake Road with Fr. Edwin Fredrick as celebrant. Burial will be in Grand Traverse Memorial Gardens.

A rosary will be recited Monday at 8 p.m. at the Reynolds funeral home.

Memorials may be directed to the Carmelite Monastery, Silver Lake Road.

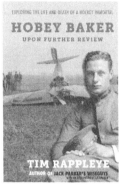

HOBEY BAKER: UPON FURTHER REVIEW
Exploring the Life and Death of a Hockey Immortal
By Tim Rappleye

He was America's most dashing athlete, the pride of Princeton. Hobey Baker, the aristocratic Ivy League sports hero and, later, a glamorous World War I fighter pilot. From the outside, U.S. Army Captain Hobey Baker had it all: good looks, a glamorous fiancé, war medals for bravery, and a sports resume second to none. And then it all came crashing down, barely a month following the Armistice.

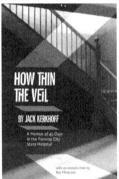

HOW THIN THE VEIL:
A Memoir of 45 Days in the Traverse City State Hospital
By Jack Kerkhoff
with an introduction by Ray Minervini
How Thin the Veil is a 45-day account of Kerkhoff's treatment, his conversations with the nurses and doctors (some of them with their real names), his interactions with the inmates, and his trips to downtown Traverse City watering holes. There's also romance in the form of Suzy, a pretty, lisping waif whose "bad spells" had kept her hospitalized for eight years. First published in 1952, How Thin the Veil shines a "hard-boiled" light on the mid-century conditions of patients of mental illness.

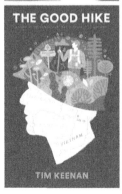

THE GOOD HIKE:
A Story of the Appalachian Trail, PTSD, and Love
By Tim Keenan
The Good Hike is the story of a journey from Georgia to Maine in the shadow of the Vietnam war. It's a story of resilience, of goodness, of camaraderie, love, and of a man trying to find peace within his post traumatic stress disorder (PTSD).

AND CHANDLER LAKE BOOKS

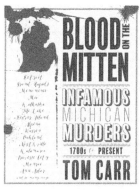

BLOOD ON THE MITTEN:
Infamous Michigan Murders, 1700s to Present
By Tom Carr
In this hugely effective debut, Tom Carr sheds keen illumination upon a regional inventory of killers, kooks, cutthroats and the aggressively unhinged. The tales are horrific and humorous by turns — grisly, goofy, poignant dispatches expertly summated by a skilled veteran reporter who's no stranger to the back stairs habituated by a true sleuth. Story telling at its fully imagined best."
— Ben Hamper, bestselling author of *Rivethead*

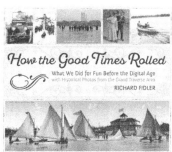

HOW THE GOOD TIMES ROLLED:
What We Did Before the Digital Age
By Richard Fidler
Believe it or not, a hundred years ago, people connected directly, face-to-face, for fun and friendship. Dozens of archival photos from the Grand Traverse Area.

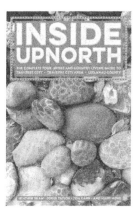

INSIDE UPNORTH:
The Complete Tour, Sport and Country Living Guide to Traverse City, Traverse City Area and Leelanau County
By Heather Shaw, Jodee Taylor, Tom Carr and many others
Whether you're planning a visit, are new to the area or you've lived here your whole life, INSIDE UPNORTH is an indispensable go-to road map to all things wonderful in Northwest Michigan.

MORE FROM MISSION POINT PRESS

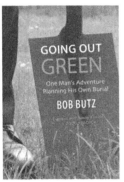

GOING OUT GREEN:
One Man's Adventure Planning His Own Natural Burial
by Bob Butz

Bob Butz, investigative reporter, humorist, and amateur naturalist is on assignment: He's planning his own natural burial in three months.

"At once elegant and funny as hell, Bob Butz has written the most useful book I've seen all year. Everyone will be needing this book. No exceptions. See you at sunset." — Doug Peacock, author of *Grizzly Years: In Search of the American Wilderness*

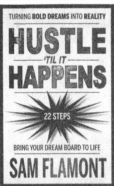

HUSTLE 'TIL IT HAPPENS:
Turning Bold Dreams Into Reality
By Sam Flamont

"Hustle 'Til It Happens provides great guidance, and the right amount of motivation, to help anyone define their goals, develop the disciplines to achieve them, and recognize that they have the power within themselves to make their dreams a reality. If you're feeling stuck, or not living the life you wanted to live, pick up this book and start taking action today." — Angie Morgan, *New York Times* Best Selling author of *Spark: How to Lead Yourself and Others to Greater Success and Leading from the Front*

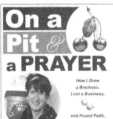

ON A PIT AND A PRAYER:
How I Grew a Business, Lost a Business, and Found Faith, Family and Love
By Michelle White

"This is a great read for any small business owner or aspiring small business owner. Many perils await in the mine field that is small business ownership, and Michelle survived them all. She takes us on a journey of passion, heart, loss and love. We have much to learn from her experiences!" — Cammie Buehler,
Managing Partner, Epicure Catering & Cherry Basket Farm

AND CHANDLER LAKE BOOKS

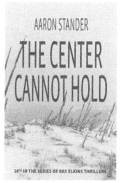

THE CENTER CANNOT HOLD

By Aaron Stander

In the depths of winter, Cedar County is on occasion literally frozen in place. Roads are impassable; the area schools are closed for days at a time. And the bad guys and gals, they're hunkered down like everyone else until the weather breaks. But this winter isn't the usual. There's arson and murder. The iniquities of some particularly unsavory ancestors are being visited upon the current generation.

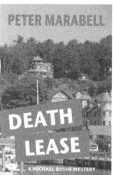
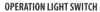

DEATH LEASE

By Peter Marabell

In 1922, Augustus Sanderson hired Charles W. Caskey, architect of Grand Hotel, to build a "majestic cottage" high on the East Bluff of Mackinac Island. Camille Sanderson, like her ancestors, assumed responsibility for the cottage when her turn came. Camille turns to private investigator Michael Russo when her ex-husband steals the lease. So begins a journey awash in deception, forgery, murder and lies.

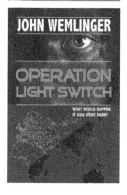

OPERATION LIGHT SWITCH

By John Wemlinger

"John Wemlinger has written a fast-moving and compelling story of overcoming a grave injustice with the help of family, friends, caring military professionals, and sheer guts."
— Ron Christmas, Lieutenant General, USMC (Ret)

"Wemlinger gets it. The nimbleness of our armed forces is as important today as its fire power. *Operation Light Switch* is a great read. Enjoyed it from cover to cover." — Mike Kelleher, Brigadier General, US Army (Ret)

Made in the USA
Monee, IL
01 August 2020